The Effective Management of Colorectal Cancer

Second edition

The Effective Management of Colorectal Cancer

Second edition

Edited by

David Cunningham MD FRCP

*Consultant Medical Oncologist, and Head of the GI and Lymphoma Units,
The Royal Marsden Hospital NHS Trust, London and Sutton, Surrey, UK*

Clare Topham FRCR

*Consultant Clinical Oncologist, St Luke's Cancer Centre,
The Royal Surrey County Hospital, Guildford, Surrey, UK*

Andrew Miles MSc MPhil PhD
*Professor of Public Health Policy and UK Key Advances Series Organiser,
University of East London, UK*

**UeL University Centre for
Public Health Policy &
Health Services Research**

**Royal College
of
Radiologists**

**Association
of
Cancer Physicians**

AESCULAPIUS MEDICAL PRESS
LONDON SAN FRANCISCO SYDNEY

Published by

Aesculapius Medical Press (London, San Francisco, Sydney)
Centre for Public Health Policy and Health Services Research
School of Health Sciences
University of East London
33 Shore Road, London E9 7TA, UK

First published 2002

British Library Cataloguing in Publication Data
A catalogue record for this book is available from the British Library

ISBN 1 903044 23 5

While the advice and information in this book are believed to be true and accurate at the
time of going to press, neither the authors nor the publishers nor the sponsoring institutions
can accept any legal responsibility or liability for any errors or omissions that may be made.
In particular (but without limiting the generality of the preceding disclaimer) every effort
has been made to check drug usages; however, it is possible that errors have been missed.
Furthermore, dosage schedules are constantly being revised and new side effects recognised.
For these reasons, the reader is strongly urged to consult the drug companies' printed
instructions before administering any of the drugs recommended in this book.

Further copies of this volume are available from:
Claudio Melchiorri
Research Dissemination Fellow
Centre for Public Health Policy and Health Services Research
School of Health Sciences
University of East London
33 Shore Road, London E9 7TA, UK

Fax: 020 8525 8661
email: claudio@keyadvances4.demon.co.uk

Typeset, printed and bound in Britain
Peter Powell Origination and Print Limited

Contents

Contributors

D Alan Anthoney PhD MRCP, Senior Lecturer in GI Oncology, University of Leeds at Cookridge Hospital, Leeds

Wendy S Atkin MPH PhD, Reader in Epidemiology, Imperial College School of Medicine and Deputy Director, Colorectal Cancer Unit, St Mark's Hospital, Harrow, Middlesex

Peter Boyle PhD FRSE, Director, Division of Epidemiology and Biostatistics, European Institute of Oncology, Milan, Italy

Gina Brown MRCP FRCR, Consultant Clinical Oncologist, The Royal Marsden Hospital NHS Trust, Sutton, Surrey

Trevor Cole MB ChB FRCP, Consultant in Clinical and Cancer Genetics, West Midlands Regional Genetics Service, Clinical Genetics Unit, Birmingham Women's Hospital, Birmingham

Colin Coles PhD, Honorary Research Professor, School of Education, King Alfred's College, Winchester, Hampshire

Brian G Ellis MB BS, General Practitioner and Senior Lecturer in General Practice, School of Postgraduate Medicine, Queen Alexandra Hospital, Portsmouth

Lynn Faulds Wood MA DipEd, Consultant for 'Beating Bowel Cancer', Twickenham

Robert Hardy BSc MB ChB FRCS, Wellcome Trust Clinical Research Fellow, Departments of Surgery and Medicine, University of Birmingham

Bill Heald OBE MChir FRCS, Professor of Surgery, University of Southampton, and Director of Surgery, North Hampshire Hospital, Basingstoke

Iona Heath MB BS, General Practitioner, Kaversham Group Practice, London

Mark Hill MD MRCP, Consultant Medical Oncologist, GI Unit, Royal Marsden NHS Trust, Sutton, Surrey

Daniel Hochhauser DPhil MRCP, Senior Lecturer in Medical Oncology, Royal Free and University Hospital, Medical School, Royal Free Hospital, London

Michael Langman BSc MD FRCP FMedSci, Professor of Medicine, Department of Medicine, University of Birmingham at Queen Elizabeth Hospital, Birmingham

Paul Mainwaring MB BS FRACP, Consultant Medical Oncologist, St Thomas' Hospital NHS Trusts, London

Nick Maisey MB BS MRCP, Specialist Registrar in Medical Oncology, GI Unit, Royal Marsden NHS Trust, Sutton, Surrey

Ceri J Phillips PhD, Health Economist, Centre for Health Economics and Policy Studies, University of Wales, Swansea

David Sebag-Montefiore FRCP FRCR, Consultant and Honorary Senior Lecturer in Clinical Oncology, Leeds Cancer Centre, Cookridge Hospital, Leeds

Matthew T Seymour MA MD MRCP, Senior Lecturer in Medical Oncology, University of Leeds at Cookridge Hospital, Leeds

H Vicky Sleightholme BSc, Cancer Co-ordinator, West Midlands Family Cancer Strategy, Clinical Genetics Unit, Birmingham Women's Hospital, Birmingham

Edwin T Swarbrick MD FRCP, Consultant Gastroenterologist, New Cross Hospital, Wolverhampton

Michael R Thompson MD FRCS, Consultant Colorectal Surgeon, Department of Surgery, Queen Alexandra Hospital, Portsmouth

Christopher Weiner MB ChB MPH, Specialist Registrar in Public Health Medicine, Institute of Public Health and Epidemiology, University of Birmingham

Preface

Colorectal cancer (CRC) incidence rates in the UK are among the highest in the world. Examination of these data from England and Wales shows marked divergences in incidence trends over the past 20 years between younger and older people and, although incidence rates have nearly halved in younger individuals, they have risen markedly in those who are older, with similar patterns being seen for cancer of the colon and rectum. Such findings emphasise the need for the early identification of individuals at risk. A proper understanding of molecular events initiating and promoting cancer development is becoming increasingly important in identifying high-risk groups for cancer screening, in determining which subgroups of patients with increased risk are most likely to develop cancer, in diagnosing cancer when histological methods are not sufficiently sensitive or specific and in developing therapy at a molecular level against tumours. More is known about the molecular basis of CRC than that of any other cancer as a result of the existence of well-characterised genetic syndromes predisposing to CRC and the fact that both sporadic and inherited cancers often develop from premalignant lesions that are amenable to biopsy and molecular analysis. It is widely accepted that active case identification and intervention is justified in familial adenomatous polyposis (FAP), given that without intervention almost 100% of carriers develop colon or rectal cancer. Accumulating evidence suggests that colonoscopic surveillance and predictive molecular testing, rather than family history analysis alone, may also be justified for hereditary non-polyposis colon cancer (HNPCC), where similar impacts on morbidity and mortality may be achievable. In addition, so-called 'lesser' family histories are also associated with the risk of CRC and the potential to detect and remove premalignant polyps is compelling for active surveillance in this larger but less well-defined group of individuals. The clinical effectiveness and cost-effectiveness of such an approach remain, however, unclear, although in the UK studies are currently under way that aim to address this issue by evaluating faecal occult blood testing (FOBT) and flexible sigmoidoscopy (FS). Part 1 comprehensively reviews currently available data on the epidemiology of colorectal cancer, the molecular basis of risk factors for the development of disease, and how these can be employed in early detection of premalignancy and malignancy through clinical genetic analysis and screening.

It is now generally accepted that the administration of 5-fluorouracil (5FU)-based chemotherapy to medically fit patients with resected node-positive colon cancer is associated with a measurable survival benefit, although the situation in node-negative disease is less clear and the value of adjuvant chemotherapy more contentious. The treatment of advanced disease remains, however, palliative with first-line therapy providing a survival benefit of approximately one year. Second-line therapy has also been shown to confer survival benefit, despite relatively low objective response rates.

For years, fluoropyrimidines have remained pivotal in the treatment of metastatic disease with many studies addressing the optimum regimen for delivery of these drugs. Indeed, different methods of their administration confer differing benefits and toxicities, and analysis of infusional schedules of 5FU/folinic acid (FA) in advanced CRC has been reported to be associated with improved survival. Indeed, in combination with the new agents oxaliplatin and irinotecan – which have modest activity when employed as single agents – high response rates with manageable toxicities are routinely achieved. The oral fluoropyrimidines capecitabine and UFT are now licensed and have the potential to replace intravenous 5FU, thus making treatment much easier for patients. Recent trials have reported similar response rates and survival for oral drugs when compared with intravenous 5FU and leucovorin. It appears likely that the use of oral fluoropyrimidines as part of combination approaches will maximise therapeutic efficacy while minimising toxicity to provide the ideal therapeutic index for patients with advanced CRC. Nevertheless, the disease remains only moderately chemosensitive and new approaches to treatment, rather than representing antimetabolites or DNA-damaging agents, are increasingly focusing on our knowledge of the biology of the disease and the inhibition of targets identified by insights into molecular pathways. Part 2 of this text reviews the current science and opinion underpinning medical intervention in the adjuvant and metastatic settings and describes current thinking and progress in relation to the development and use of novel agents.

For almost 20 years the concept of total mesorectal excision (TME) has featured in the medical literature. It remains, however, the object of ongoing controversy and sometimes of downright antagonism, probably on account of the size of the benefit claimed and also, perhaps, because of a reluctance to accept that recurrence may be the result in many cases of inadequate surgical techniques. At the time of writing, major trials are under way which are set to evaluate the technique systematically in large patient cohorts and Chapter 9 provides a thorough review of current thinking on its benefits and limitations, whether as a single surgical procedure or in combination with other treatment modalities. Indeed, there is growing evidence that preoperative radiotherapy and TME have an additive effect on improvement of local recurrence rates and there is evidence that preoperative radiotherapy or chemoradiotherapy for 'good' prognosis patients may represent over-treatment, which not only places an excessive demand on resources and is costly, but most importantly leads to significant morbidity. Thus, local staging for patient selection becomes an important factor in effective management. There is a rapidly expanding number of published studies on the use of concurrent chemoradiotherapy (CRT) in rectal cancer, the majority of which use preoperative radiotherapy where the interpretation or their results is problematic. Certainly, there are many potential end-points for studies of CRT. Phase I studies should still focus on determining the maximum tolerated dose on the basis of dose-limiting toxicity and allow a recommended schedule for phase II studies. The dose escalation could, however, be either a new drug or the dose of radiotherapy. In locally advanced rectal cancer, potential end-points as a measure of efficacy could include local recurrence, curative resection, histologically confirmed curative resection, histopathological complete response, histopathological downstaging, sphincter preservation, organ preservation and surgical complications. Part 3 provides a thorough review of the place of total mesorectal excision, the clinical effectiveness and cost-effectiveness of preoperative staging, and the value of chemoradiotherapy in rectal cancer.

Part 4, the final part, discusses current NHS health policy in relation to the clinical significance and biological reasoning underpinning the '2-week wait'. The Government introduced this policy because some patients with CRC had unacceptably long delays waiting for an outpatient appointment, and the Department of Health asked the Association of Coloproctology of Great Britain and Ireland, the British Society for Gastroenterology and the Royal College of General Practitioners to provide referral guidelines for general practitioners. Agreed, the efficient management of all patients with lower gastrointestinal symptoms is the key to effective management of the few patients who were later confirmed to have CRC, but it is argued that the introduction of the 2-week wait standard will do little to solve the fundamental problem of the inadequacy of resources available to the clinicians who investigate and manage this disease. Indeed, estimates of the cost of personnel to run diagnostic clinics indicate that these will have to include nurse and GP endoscopists as well as gastrointestinal physicians and surgeons.

In the current age, where doctors and health professionals are increasingly overwhelmed by clinical information, we have aimed to provide a fully current, fully referenced text which is as succinct as possible, but as comprehensive as necessary. Consultants in gastroenterology and surgical, clinical and medical oncology and their trainees are likely to find it of particular use as part of their continuing professional development and specialist training, respectively, and we advance it explicitly as an excellent tool for these purposes. The book will also, we anticipate, function well as a reference volume for clinical nurse specialists and oncology pharmacists and should prove of singular use to commissioners of health services and policy makers as the basis of discussion and negotiation of health contracts with their practising colleagues.

In conclusion we thank Bristol-Myers Squibb (Oncology) Ltd for the grant of educational sponsorship which helped organise a national symposium held with The Royal College of Radiologists and Association of Cancer Physicians at The Royal College of Physicians of London, at which synopses of the constituent chapters of this book were presented.

David Cunningham MD FRCP
Clare Topham FRCR
Andrew Miles MSc MPhil PhD

Acknowledgements

The following colleagues contributed as members of the expert planning committee for the year 2000 colorectal cancer key advances project: Dr Gina Brown, Dr David Cunningham, Dr Mark Hill, Professor Roger James, Professor Andrew Miles, Dr David Sebag-Montefiore, Dr Matt Seymour and Dr Clare Topham. The contribution of Dr Andreas Polychronis, Specialist Registrar in Medical Oncology, St George's Hospital, London, as secretary to the committee and assistant editor in the preparation of the current volume, is also acknowledged.

PART 1

Epidemiology, genetics and screening

Chapter 1

Colorectal cancer epidemiology

Michael Langman and Peter Boyle

Introduction

Colorectal cancer is a common disease throughout developed communities. The bases are mainly likely to be environmental. Increases in risk are generally found in people who smoke and drink alcohol. Risk is also associated with animal protein intake and, possibly, fat intake, although reduced risk is detectable in those consuming larger quantities of fruit and vegetables.

There is limited knowledge about the specific factors responsible. Folate appears to be protective and folate intake may modulate alcohol-associated risks. Much evidence also indicates that non-steroidal anti-inflammatory drug intake reduces risk, as does hormone replacement therapy in women; calcium and vitamin D intake may also be protective. Trials of strategies designed to reduce risk through diminishing the occurrence of precursor polyp occurrence, e.g. with antioxidant regimens, have so far been disappointing.

Colorectal cancer is the most common form of digestive cancer in most developed countries. In England and Wales there are over 25,000 cases diagnosed each year, and it is the second most common form of cancer in both men and women.

Incidence

Disease frequency increases steadily with age, and Table 1.1 shows mean age-specific incidence data for the years 1990–92 for England and Wales (Cancer Statistics Registration 1995, 1997, 1999). Although rates increase in both men and women, there is a tendency for rates in men to be proportionately higher than in women with increasing age after early middle age. The reasons for this pattern are unclear. The possibilities include a greater impact of specific causal factors in men with advancing age, and a greater tendency of women to receive diagnostic procedures that reveal precursor lesions in older age groups. In keeping with this possibility is evidence that the chances of survival tend to be greater in women than in men. Table 1.2 shows some comparative standardised data for age in selected countries with high incidence rates (Boyle & Langman 2001). These indicate that within developed countries high incidences can be found in various racial groups, and that the underlying bases almost certainly reflect environmental factors.

Table 1.1 Age-specific incidence rates of colonic and rectal cancer in England and Wales, 1990–92 per 100,000 per year in men and women aged 40–74 years (Cancer Statistics Registration 1995, 1997, 1999)

Age (years)	Colon		Rectum	
	M	F	M	F
40–	7.0	6.9	4.8	3.9
45–	11.9	12.8	11.3	7.7
50–	26.2	24.0	24.1	13.6
55–	44.0	38.6	76.1	61.2
60–	76.1	61.2	61.3	31.4
65–	117.6	91.1	90.1	46.0
70–	159.6	122.9	121.3	59.3

Table 1.2 Age-standardised incidence of colorectal cancer in North America and Europe in 1988–92 in men per 100,000 per year (Boyle & Langman 2001)

Asia and Australasia:	
Australia (New South Wales)	46.9
Japan (Hiroshima) (1988–90)	50.9
Europe:	
Czech Republic	48.2
France (Haut Rhin)	49.9
Italy (Trieste)	49.4
North America:	
Canada:	
Nova Scotia	47.8
Newfoundland	47.3
USA:	
US Hawaii (Japanese)	53.5
Detroit: black	48.3
San Francisco: black	47.9

Adapted from Parkin *et al.* (1997).

Time trends

Incidence rates, taken overall, in the UK have been rising steadily for the last 20 years. This is unlikely to be explained by more efficient ascertainment in recent years, and causal factors must be presumed to have become more pronounced. The remaining possibility – less attention to precursor lesions – seems implausible. By contrast, mortality rates have not tended to rise in the same way or have even fallen. Both pieces of evidence taken together suggest that treatment success has improved. How much any improvement is the result of detection of earlier disease and how much of better treatment is unclear.

Social factors

Smoking

Although evidence conflicts (Baron *et al.* 1994; Giovannucci *et al.* 1994a; Heinemann *et al.* 1994), there appears to be a suggestion of a modest increase in risk in people who smoke for both colon and rectal cancer. For reasons that are unclear, the risk of benign polyps seems to be more consistently increased in those who smoke (Kikendall *et al.* 1989; Kearney *et al.* 1995). This is rather weak evidence to indicate that, if the effect is direct, it may operate fairly early in cancer induction. As with carcinoma of the oesophagus, separation from the effects of alcohol is difficult. However, data collected prospectively in the Nurses Health Study and the Health Professionals Follow-up Study in the USA and elsewhere have indicated that there are likely to be independent contributory factors from smoking, alcohol and low folate intake (Giovannucci *et al.* 1993; Baron *et al.* 1998), which contribute to raised risk of developing hyperplastic colon polyps. These same factors also seem to be associated with the well-defined precursor lesions for colorectal cancer – adenomatous polyps – and with colorectal cancer itself.

Alcohol

Moderate increases in risk are seen in people who drink alcohol (Stemmermann *et al.* 1990; Kune & Vinetta 1992). Trends are more consistent and more obvious than for smoking, and cannot be removed by adjusting for smoking habits. It is unclear if any effect is direct, or whether it reflects removal of folate in alcohol handling, thus making the vitamin unavailable for cancer prevention (see below).

Diet

The unequivocal demonstration that dietary constituents influence liability to colorectal cancer, as with other cancers, is difficult. Retrospective dietary enquiries are subject to unquantifiable biases caused by knowledge of who are patients and who are controls, and to changing perception over periods long past about the characteristics of diet at that time. Prospective studies are inevitably harder to mount, take many years to come to fruition, and still have the problems associated with determining whether an association of a particular nutrient with liability to cancer actually reflects a close and direct relationship, or is better explained indirectly by another factor. Examination of the physical characteristics of individuals who develop colorectal cancer has given inconsistent evidence of prior obesity. It has also shown inconsistent or no evidence of raised serum cholesterol levels at periods in the lives of patients before any illness related to the cancer would be likely to have impacted on the findings (Chute *et al.* 1991; Chyou *et al.* 1994; Giovannucci *et al.* 1995a). Such features might suggest that dietary fat intake may not turn out to be a dominant risk-associated factor.

Fat

Fat, particularly animal fat, is a major constituent of the Western diet. Examination of major nutrient intakes has contrasted those of fat, particularly animal fat, and protein, with fruit and vegetables. There are possible mechanistic bases for considering all three separately. Thus dietary fat intake could alter patterns of bile salt secretion and hence the concentrations of bile acids to which the colonic epithelium is exposed, possibly through favouring the establishment of one or another bacterial population. Enquiries into fat intake levels have generally shown rather modest correlations with risks of colon cancer or benign polyps (Sandler *et al.* 1993; Giovannucci *et al.* 1994b; Chyou *et al.* 1996).

Protein

Altered protein intake could influence hepatic microsomal activity, so altering the concentrations of metabolised procarcinogens in the body, or carcinogens could be produced when meat is charred during cooking. Effects favouring particular intraintestinal bacterial flora are also possible. Better correlations have sometimes been found between protein intakes from animal sources and large intestinal cancer or polyp risks than for fat (Potter & McMichael 1986; Giovannucci *et al.* 1994b), although sometimes attenuated by allowing for other nutrients. On the other hand, others have found better inverse correlations with carbohydrate intake (Sandler *et al.* 1993; Kearney *et al.* 1995) and an unexpected increase in risk detected for sucrose-containing foods (Bostick *et al.* 1994), with none for protein in individuals developing hyperplastic polyps (Kearney *et al.* 1995).

Fibre intake

Colorectal cancer incidence is, generally, higher in industrialised countries with a Western lifestyle, with disease incidence tending to be greater in those who are overweight. In the past, parallels have been drawn among rising incidences of appendicitis, diverticular disease and colonic cancer, suggesting that the common factor is low dietary fibre intake in the Western diet. However, the parallel has diminished as the frequency of appendicitis has fallen, whereas colon cancer incidence has risen. Furthermore, there is the need to consider the many sources of dietary fibre, whether from fruit, vegetables or cereals.

Fruit and vegetables

Apart from providing vitamin C, an antioxidant, fruit and vegetables also provide folate which is of central importance in supplying methyl groups which could have considerable influences, among other properties, through methylating and silencing DNA. Epidemiological evidence shows, reasonably in some (Chute *et al.* 1991; Chyou *et al.* 1996) but not other (Kearney *et al.* 1995; Giovannucci *et al.* 1995a) studies, that higher intakes of fruit and vegetables are associated with protection from colonic cancer, and also from colonic polyps, and further data indicate that folate may be the, or an, important factor (Benito *et al.* 1991; Freudenheim *et al.* 1991; Ferraroni *et al.* 1994; Bird *et al.* 1995). Consistent with this evidence, alcohol consumption, which increases the demand for folate, is also associated with increased risks (Stemmermann *et al.* 1990; Kune & Vinetta 1992). Effects of folate are likely to be direct because depletion raises the susceptibility of rodents to large bowel carcinogens, and repletion lowers the risk (Cravo *et al.* 1992; Kim *et al.* 1996).

It has been suggested that folate is beneficial because, by acting as a methyl donor through its metabolite 5,10-methyltetrahydrofolate (THF) in methylating homocysteine, it raises the amount of methionine available to methylate DNA through the intermediary *S*-adenosyl-methionine (SAM), and so protects against mutagens by stabilising histones (Bestor 1998).

Chemoprevention

Non-steroidal anti-inflammatory drugs and aspirin

The observation that those who take non-steroidal anti-inflammatory drugs (NSAIDs) are at reduced risk of colorectal cancer has been confirmed repeatedly (Logan *et al.* 1993; Peleg *et al.* 1994; Giovannucci *et al.* 1995b). Support for direct effects includes evidence that cyclo-oxygenase (COX) type 2 is upregulated in colonic tumours with more consistent rises in carcinomas than in adenomas, and that NSAIDs protect against experimental colonic carcinogenesis and induce programmed cell death, or inhibit growth in colon cancer cell lines (Reddy *et al.* 1993; Hixson *et al.* 1994; Shiff *et al.* 1995). Patients with familial polyposis coli develop fewer and smaller polyps than expected when treated with NSAIDs (Giardiello *et al.* 1993; Hirota *et al.* 1996). Doses required seem to be in the ordinary therapeutic range. In keeping with evidence that COX-2 is upregulated (Eberhart *et al.* 1994) are results that suggest that selective COX-2 antagonists may be as effective as non-selective antagonists in inhibiting colon cancer cell growth (Sheng *et al.* 1997), that COX-2 is upregulated in carcinogen-induced animal tumours (Dubois *et al.* 1996), and that knock-out of the gene inhibits polyp formation in mice genetically prone to develop polyps (Oshima *et al.* 1996). That effects may not wholly arise through COX antagonism is suggested by evidence for protection from sulindac sulphide, which is not, for practical purposes, a COX inhibitor. Observational data suggest that full, as opposed to cardiopreventive, doses of aspirin may be required to prevent cancer development in humans. Overall risk reduction may be of the order of 30–40% for both cancer and adenoma; estimates tend to be higher when derived from retrospective case–control studies than from data obtained in large long-term population studies. Risk reduction is unlikely to be unique to colorectal cancer, and parallel falls in incidence may be seen for gastric and oesophageal cancer (Langman *et al.* 2000).

Hormone replacement therapy

Women who take oestrogens postmenopausally are at reduced risk of colorectal cancer (Calle *et al.* 1995; Newcomb & Storer 1995). Reductions in rates are of the order of a third, as with NSAIDs. Mechanisms are unclear. However, oestrogen receptors are demonstrable in colonic mucosa (Singh *et al.* 1993), particularly β-receptors, and are presumably functional. But so far it has been difficult to find evidence that oestrogens have substantial effects on the growth of tumour cell lines, and treatment with the anti-oestrogen, tamoxifen, has not seemed to influence the behaviour of large bowel tumours in humans. A further indicator of functional response to oestrogen in the colon is, however, that aromatase and a 17β-steroid dehydrogenase are easily demonstrable in colonic mucosa, and appear to be responsible for oestrone–estradiol shifts (English *et al.* 1999). Although most epidemiological studies suggest that use of hormone replacement therapy (HRT) is associated with protection against colonic cancer, evidence is not completely in favour, and doubt about the evidence suggesting protection by oestrogen could be increased by data that indicate that oral contraceptive use does not appear to be protective. Such a discrepancy may be explained by lack of difference in premenopausal women between normal physiological hormonal exposure and substituted pharmacological doses.

Studies of the possible protective effects associated with the use of HRT have been carried out in women with a wide variety of ages. Most have been at least 50, and have here suggested protection. However, it is noteworthy that one study, conducted in individuals in their 40s, showed no evidence of protection. It can be argued that these women, who had until relatively recently been exposed to normal oestrogenic and progestogenic hormonal environments, might not be a satisfactory group in whom to seek evidence of protection by HRT, or at least until any putative protective effects had worn off. A possible set of mechanisms lies in the existence of functional oestrogen receptors in the colon, but so far it has been difficult to find evidence that oestrogens have substantial effects on the growth of tumour cell lines and treatment with the anti-oestrogen, tamoxifen, has not seemed to influence the behaviour of large bowel tumours in humans. There is, however, some evidence that use of HRT is associated with reduction in blood homocysteine levels, so that it is possible that at least part of any effect of HRT in influencing the frequency of colonic cancer is through altering DNA methylation.

Micronutrients

The relevance of micronutrients to the development of colorectal cancer can be explored by reference to data exploring possible epidemiological associations, and by consideration of the influence of deliberate dietary supplementation in the modulation of polyp incidence, as well as by examining the findings in animal studies (Langman & Boyle 1998).

Vitamins A, C and E

Although one moderate-sized trial suggested protection against adenoma formation, another that is almost three times as large was negative (Roncucci *et al.* 1993; Greenberg *et al.* 1994). The general place in treatment of vitamin A and its analogues has been called into question by the finding, in three large randomised controlled trials, that individuals at high risk of lung cancer who receive vitamin A may be at raised rather than lowered risk of the disease (Alpha-Tocopherol, Beta-Carotene Cancer Prevention Study Group 1994; Hennekens & Buring 1996; Omenn *et al.* 1996). This evidence is backed by colon cancer cell culture studies which indicate that retinoids can interfere with the suppression of cell multiplication; these can be affected by vitamin D (Kane *et al.* 1996).

Vitamin D and calcium

Exposure to sunlight appears to be geographically associated with reduced risk of colonic cancer (Emerson & Weiss 1992), and serum vitamin D levels inversely related to risk (Garland *et al.* 1989). That such relationships are direct is indicated by evidence that vitamin D receptors are demonstrable in the colon; in addition, low concentrations of vitamin D, of the levels found in plasma, reduce the multiplication rate of colon cancer cell lines (Kane *et al.* 1994, 1996). Whether actions are through modulation of calcium ion concentrations is unclear. Other lines of evidence indicate that the oral intake of calcium salts could also have beneficial effects (Langman & Boyle 1998). Analogues of vitamin D with greatly reduced effects on calcium concentrations have been synthesised, and an analogue is already clinically available for the treatment of psoriasis, in which it reduces skin epithelial cell turnover.

Folate

The promising evidence suggesting that some, if not all, of any protective effect of diets rich in fruit and vegetables can be attributed to their folate content has been referred to earlier.

References

Alpha-Tocopherol, Beta-carotene Cancer Prevention Study Group (1994). The effect of vitamin E and beta-carotene on the incidence of lung cancer and other cancers in male smokers. *New England Journal of Medicine* **330**, 1029–1035

Baron JA, Gerhardsson de Verdier M, Ekbom A (1994). Coffee, tea, tobacco, and cancer of the large bowel. *Cancer Epidemiology, Biomarkers and Prevention* **3**, 565–570

Baron JA, Sandler RS, Haile RW, Mandel JS, Mott LA, Greenberg ER (1998). Folate intake, alcohol consumption, cigarette smoking, and risk of colorectal adenomas. *Journal of the National Cancer Institute* **90**, 57–62

Benito E, Stiggelbout A, Bosch FX *et al.* (1991). Nutritional factors in colorectal cancer risk: a case-control study in Majorca. *International Journal of Cancer* **49**, 161–167

Bestor TH (1998). Methylation meets acetylation. *Nature* **393**, 311–312

Bird CL, Swendseid ME, Witte JS *et al.* (1995). Red cell and plasma folate, folate consumption, and the risk of colorectal adenomatous polyps. *Cancer Epidemiology, Biomarkers and Prevention* **4**, 709–714

Bostick RH, Potter JD, Kushi LH *et al.* (1994). Sugar, meat and fat intake, and non-dietary risk factors for colon cancer incidence in Iowa women (United States). *Cancer Causes and Control* **5**, 38–52

Boyle P & Langman MJS (2001). Epidemiology. In Kerr DJ, Young AM, Hobbs FDR (eds) *ABC of Colorectal Cancer*. London: BMJ Books

Calle E, Miracle, Mahill HL *et al.* (1995). Estrogen replacement therapy and risk of fatal colon cancer in a prospective cohort of postmenopausal women. *Journal of the National Cancer Institute* **87**, 517–523

Cancer Statistics Registration (1995). *Office for National Statistics*. Series MB1 No. 23. London: HMSO

Cancer Statistics Registration (1997). *Office for National Statistics*. Series MB1 No. 24. London: HMSO

Cancer Statistics Registration (1999). *Office for National Statistics*. Series MB1 No. 25. London: HMSO

Chute CG, Willett WC, Colditz GA *et al.* (1991). A prospective study of body mass, height and smoking on the risk of colorectal cancer in women. *Cancer Causes Control* **2**, 117–124

Chyou PH, Nomura AM, Stemmermann GN (1994). A prospective study of weight, body mass index and other anthropometric measurements in relation to site-specific cancers. *International Journal of Cancer* **57**, 313–317

Chyou PH, Nomura AM, Stemmermann GN (1996). A prospective study of colon and rectal cancer among Hawaii Japanese men. *Annals of Epidemiology* **6**, 276–282

Cravo ML, Mason JB, Dayal Y *et al.* (1992). Folate deficiency enhances the development of colonic neoplasia in dimethylhydrazine-treated rats. *Cancer Research* **52**, 5002–5006

Dubois R, Radhika A, Reddy BS *et al.* (1996). Increased cyclooxygenase-2 gene level in carcinogen-induced rat colonic tumors. *Gastroenterology* **110**, 1259

Eberhart CE, Coffey RJ, Radhika A *et al.* (1994). Upregulation of cyclooxygenase-2 gene expression in human colorectal adenomas and adenocarcinomas. *Gastroenterology* **107**, 1183

Emerson JC & Weiss NS (1992). Colorectal cancer and solar irradiation. *Cancer Causes and Control* **3**, 95–99

English MA, Kane KF, Cruikshank N, Langman MJS, Stewart PM, Hewison M (1999). loss of estrogen inactivation in colonic cancer. *Journal of Clinical Endocrinology and Metabolism* **84**, 2080–2085

Ferraroni M, La Vecchia C, D'Avanzo B, Negri E, Franceschi S, Decarli A (1994). Selected micronutrient intake and the risk of colorectal cancer. *British Journal of Cancer* **70**, 1150–1155

Freudenheim JL, Graham S, Marshall JR, Haughey BP, Cholewinski S, Wilkinson G (1991). Folate intake and carcinogenesis of the colon and rectum. *International Journal of Epidemiology* **20**, 368–374

Garland CF, Comstock GW, Garland GW *et al.* (1989). Serum 25-hydroxyvitamin D and colon cancer: eight year prospective study. *The Lancet* **ii**, 1176–1178.

Giardiello FM, Hamilton SR, Krush AJ *et al.* (1993). Treatment of colonic and rectal adenomas with sulindac in familial adenomatous polyposis. *New England Journal of Medicine* **328**, 1313

Giovannucci E, Stampfer MJ, Colditz GA *et al*. (1993). Folate, methionine, and alcohol intake and risk of colorectal adenoma. *Journal of the National Cancer Institute* **85**, 875–884

Giovannucci E, Rimm EB, Stampfer MJ *et al*. (1994a). A prospective study of cigarette smoking and risk of colorectal adenoma and colorectal cancer in U.S. men. *Journal of the National Cancer Institute* **86**, 183–191

Giovannucci E, Rimm EB, Stampfer MJ, Colditz GA, Ascherio A, Willett WC (1994b). Intake of fat, meat and fiber in relation to risk colon cancer in men. *Cancer Research* **54**, 2390–2397

Giovannucci E, Ascherio A, Rimm EB, Colditz GA, Stampfer MJ, Willett WC (1995a). Physical activity, obesity, and risk for colon cancer and adenoma in men. *Annals of Internal Medicine* **122**, 327–334

Giovannucci E, Egan KM, Hunter DJ *et al*. (1995b). Aspirin and the risk of colorectal cancer in women. *New England Journal of Medicine* **333**, 609

Greenberg ER, Baron JA, Tosteson TA *et al*. (1994). A clinical trial of antioxidant vitamins to prevent colorectal adenoma. *New England Journal of Medicine* **331**, 141–147

Heinemann EF, Zahm SH, McLaughlin JK, Vaught JB (1994). Increased risk of colorectal cancer among smokers: results of a 26-year follow-up of US veterans and a review. *International Journal of Cancer* **59**, 728–738

Hennekens CH & Buring JE (1996). Long term supplementation with beta-carotene on the incidence of malignant neoplasms and cardiovascular disease. *New England Journal of Medicine* **334**, 1145–1149

Hirota C, Iida M, Aoyagi K *et al*. (1996). Effect of indomethacin suppositories on rectal polyposis in patients with familial adenomatous polyposis. *Cancer* **78**, 1660

Hixson LJ, Alberts DS, Krutzsch M *et al*. (1994). Antiproliferative effect of nonsteroidal antiinflammatory drugs against human colon cancer cells. *Cancer Epidemiology, Biomarkers and Prevention* **3**, 433

Kane KF, Langman MJS, Williams GR (1994). 1, 25-dihydroxy vitamin D3 and retinoid X receptor expression in human colorectal neoplasms. *Gut* **36**, 255–258

Kane KF, Langman MJS, Williams GR (1996). Antiproliferative responses of two human colon cancer cell lines to vitamin D3 are differentially modified by 9-*cis*-retinoic acid. *Cancer Research* 56, 623–632

Kearney J, Giovannucci E, Rimm EB *et al*. (1995). Diet, alcohol, and smoking and the occurrence of hyperplastic polyps of the colon and rectum (United States). *Cancer Causes and Control* **6**, 45–56

Kikendall JW, Bowen PE, Burgess MB, Magnetti C, Woodward J, Langenberg P (1989). Cigarettes and alcohol as independent risk factors for colonic adenomas. *Gastroenterology* **97**, 660–664

Kim YI, Salomon RN, Graeme-Cook F *et al*. (1996). Dietary folate protects against the development of macroscopic neoplasia in a dose responsive manner in rats. *Gut* **39**, 732–740

Kune GA & Vinetta L (1992). Alcohol consumption and the etiology of colorectal cancer: a review of the scientific evidence from 1957 to 1991. *Nutrition and Cancer* **18**, 97–111

Langman MJS & Boyle P (1998). Chemoprevention of colorectal cancer. *Gut* **43**, 578–585

Langman MJS, Cheng KK, Gilman EA, Lancashire RJ (2000). Effect of anti-inflammatory drugs on overall risk of common cancer: case-control study in general practice research database. *British Medical Journal* **320**, 1642–1646

Logan RFA, Little J, Hawtin PC *et al*. (1993). Effect of aspirin and non-steroidal anti-inflammatory drugs on colorectal adenomas: case-control study of subjects participating in the Nottingham faecal occult blood screening programme. *British Medical Journal* **307**, 285

Newcomb BA & Storer BE (1995). Postmenopausal hormone use and risk of large bowel cancer. *Journal of the National Cancer Institute* **87**, 1067–1071

Omenn GS, Goodman G, Thornqvist MA *et al*. (1996). Effects of combination of beta-carotene and vitamin A on lung cancer and cardiovascular disease. *New England Journal of Medicine* **334**, 1150–1155

Oshima M, Dinchuk JE, Kargman SL *et al*. (1996). Suppression of intestinal polyposis in Apc delta716 knockout mice by inhibition of cyclooxygenase 2 (Cox-2). *Cell* **87**, 803

Parkin *et al*. (1997). *Cancer Incidence in Five Continents*, Vol VII. IARC Scientific Publications

Peleg I, Maibach HT, Brown SH *et al*. (1994). Aspirin and non-steroidal anti-inflammatory drug use and the risk of subsequent colorectal cancer. *Archives of Internal Medicine* **154**, 394

Potter JD, McMichael AJ (1986). Diet and cancer of the colon and rectum: a case-control study. *Journal of the National Cancer Institute* **76**, 557–569

Reddy BS, Rao CV, Rivenson A *et al*. (1993). Inhibitory effect of aspirin on azoxymethane-induced colon carcinogenesis in rats. *Carcinogenesis* **14**, 1493

Roncucci L, Di Donato P, Carati L *et al*. (1993). Antioxidant vitamins or lactulose for the prevention of the recurrence of colorectal adenomas. *Diseases of the Colon and Rectum*. **36**, 227–234

Sandler RS, Lyles CM, Peipins LA, McAuliffe CA, Woosley JT, Kupper LL (1993). Diet and risk of colorectal adenomas: macronutrients, cholesterol, and fiber. *Journal of the National Cancer Institute* **85**, 884–891

Sheng H, Shao J, Kirkland SC *et al*. (1997). Inhibition of human colon cancer cell growth by selective inhibition of cyclooxygenase-2. *Journal of Clinical Investigation* **99**, 2254

Shiff SJ, Qiao L, Rigas B *et al*. (1995). Sulindac sulfide, an aspirin-like compound inhibits proliferation, causes cell cycle quiescence and induces apoptosis in HT-29 colon adenocarcinoma cells. *Journal of Clinical Investigation* **96**, 491

Singh S, Sheppard MC, Langman MJS *et al*. (1993). Sex differences in the incidence of colorectal cancer: an exploration of oestrogen and progesterone receptors. *Gut* **34**, 611–615

Stemmermann GN, Nomura AM, Chyou PH *et al*. (1990). Prospective study of alcohol intake and large bowel cancer. *Digestive Diseases and Sciences* **35**, 1414–1420

Molecular basis for risk factors in colorectal cancer – genetic syndromes, adenomatous colorectal polyps and ulcerative colitis

Robert Hardy

Introduction

Knowledge of the molecular basis of colorectal cancer development is better understood than that of any other malignancy. This is the result, first, of insight gained from genetic syndromes predisposing to colorectal cancer, the molecular basis of which is known and, second, the fact that both heritable and sporadic cancers usually develop from premalignant lesions that are amenable to biopsy and molecular analysis.

Understanding molecular events that initiate and promote cancer development is becoming increasingly important in five main clinical areas:

1. Identifying high-risk groups for cancer screening.
2. Determining which subgroups of patients with increased risk are most likely to develop cancer.
3. As an aid to diagnosis when histological methods are not sufficiently sensitive or specific.
4. Forming molecular profiles of tumours.
5. Tailoring treatment to individual tumours and developing therapy at a molecular level.

The most common genetic syndromes displaying an elevated colorectal cancer risk – familial adenomatous polypsis (FAP) and hereditary non-polyposis colorectal cancer (HNPCC) – account for 0.5–1% and 2–5.5% of total colorectal cancer cases, respectively. Individuals within the general population with a positive family history for colorectal cancer have themselves an approximately twofold increased risk (Woolf 1958; Lovett 1976; Bale *et al*. 1984; Burt *et al*. 1985; Carstensen *et al*. 1996). This familial clustering of colorectal cancer cases within the general population implies that the vast majority of family history-positive cancers involve genetic and epigenetic events beyond those occurring in FAP and HNPCC. Evidence is, however, lacking on particular factors associated with this increased family history risk.

Excluding classically inherited genetic syndromes, two colorectal pathologies are particularly associated with an increased cancer risk: sporadic adenomatous polyps and extensive chronic ulcerative colitis. These two lesions show both overlapping and unique patterns of oncogene, tumour-suppressor gene and epigenetic alterations, which are proposed as leading to tumour initiation and progression. Table 2.1 gives an overview of clinical and molecular correlates for FAP, attenuated FAP, HNPCC and ulcerative colitis-associated neoplasia.

Table 2.1 Clinical and molecular correlates of familial adenomatous polyposis (FAP), attenuated FAP (AFAP), hereditary non-polyposis colorectal cancer (HNPCC) and ulcerative colitis-associated neoplasia (UCAN)

	FAP	AFAP	HNPCC	UCAN
Mean age at cancer diagnosis (years)	32–39	45–55	42–29	40–70
Cancer distribution	Random	? Right-sided predominance	Mainly right colon	Influence by disease site
Number of polyps	>100	1–100	Often 1 (tumour)	Often 0
Male:female ratio	1:1	1:1	1.5:1	1:1
Endoscopic view of polyp	Pedunculated	Mainly flat	Pedunculated (45%), flat (55%)	None
Lag time from adenoma to cancer (years)	10–20	10	5	? >8
Proportion of colorectal cancer (%)	0.5–1	0.5	1–5	< 0.5
Superficial stigmata	80% retinal pigmentation	None	Only in Muir–Torre syndrome	None
Polyp distribution	Distal or universal	Mainly proximal to splenic flexure	Mainly proximal to splenic flexure	None
Carcinoma histology	Often exophytic growth	Variable	Inflammation Increased mucin	Mucosal ulceration and inflammation
Other associated tumours	Duodenal adenoma, cerebral and thyroid tumours, desmoids	Duodenal adenoma	Endometrial, ovarian, gastric, glioblastoma, many others	None
Gene (chromosome) mutation	APC (5q21) distal to 5'	APC (5q21) proximal to 5'	MSH2 (2p), MLH1 (3p21), PMS1 (2q31), PMS2 (7p22)	Multiple, including 17p(p53), 5q(APC), 9p(p16)

Adapted from Hardy et al. (2001).

This chapter aims to give a state-of-the-art overview of the known molecular basis for risk factors in colorectal cancer, with particular emphasis on how this knowledge can aid clinical decision-making in patients with a diagnosis of, or at increased risk from, this common malignancy.

Genetic instability in colorectal cancer

An understanding of the molecular changes occurring in colorectal cancer necessitates an understanding of genetic instability, a phenomenon occurring in most malignancies. Genetic instability can be subdivided into two major types: chromosomal instability (CIN) and microsatellite instability (MIN). CIN encompasses changes occurring at gene and chromosome levels, such as loss of heterozygosity, aneuploidy and chromosomal translocation. MIN is characterised by mutation in mono-, di- and trinucleotide repeats (termed 'microsatellites') within the genome, occurring as a result of defects in DNA-repair mechanisms (defective mismatch repair). Whereas CIN is a phenomenon that should show little variability in detection using molecular techniques, MIN analysis is more prone to artefact arising principally from microsatellite marker selection and the detection technique used. For this reason, studies often report varying rates of MIN when looking at similar lesions, and a classification into high and low grades of MIN seems appropriate for purposes of comparison.

Most tumours exhibit an increased background mutation rate, but it has not been established whether this in itself is sufficient for tumorigenesis, or whether selection of clones with a growth advantage is the primary mechanism for progression of malignancy (Lengauer *et al.* 1998; Tomlinson & Bodmer 1999). Furthermore, a recent study suggests that the proportion of tumours with unstable genomes may be smaller than was originally thought, and the nature and extent of mutations may be more important then their rate of acquisition (Georgiades *et al.* 1999).

Epigenetic events in colorectal cancer

Epigenetics is defined as modifications of the genome, heritable during cell division, that do not involve a change in the DNA sequence. The study of epigenetics in cancer biology has increased rapidly in recent years, driven initially by studies of DNA methylation in tumours. Global hypomethylation (Feinberg *et al.* 1988), hypomethylation of individual genes (Feinberg & Vogelstein 1983) and hypermethylation of gene promoter sequences (Baylin *et al.* 1986) have all been shown to modulate gene expression differentially in normal and tumour tissue. An example of this is *MMR* gene expression in sporadic colorectal cancer (see later).

An important example of epigenetic modifications in colorectal cancer concerns loss of imprinting (LOI). Imprinting is the process whereby expression from a paternal allele is silenced, leading to differential expression from paternally and maternally derived alleles. Loss of imprinting reverses this effect, and can lead to activation of growth-promoting imprinted genes or silencing of tumour-suppressor genes.

In colorectal cancer and, more importantly, matched normal colon mucosa, LOI has been described for insulin-like growth factor II (IGF-II) (Cui *et al*. 1998; Nakagawa *et al*. 2001). This important finding implies that individuals with LOI may have the equivalent of a 'field change', increasing susceptibility to cancer development. If such hypotheses are substantiated, screening for LOI in normal colon biopsies may stratify individuals into low- or high-risk groups.

Attention is now paid to syndromes displaying an increased risk of colorectal cancer: FAP, HNPCC, Peutz–Jeghers syndrome and hyperplastic polyposis.

Familial adenomatous polyposis

Molecular basis of FAP

The genetic basis of FAP is a germline (inherited) mutation in one allele of the adenomatous polyposis coli (*APC*) gene on chromosome 5q (Bodmer *et al*. 1987; Leppert *et al*. 1987). FAP displays autosomal dominant inheritance (Veale 1965), but may also arise from spontaneous mutation of an *APC* allele in the germline, accounting for cases with no pre-existing family history. It is generally accepted that inactivation or loss of the wild-type *APC* gene in FAP patients leads to polyp initiation. *APC* has thus been termed the 'gatekeeper' of polyp development (Kinzler & Vogelstein 1998), and mutation of this gene is indeed also the most common early event in sporadic adenoma formation (Kinzler & Vogelstein 1996). In this manner, APC acts as a tumour-suppressor gene, with inactivation of both alleles necessary for tumour initiation. There is increasing evidence, however, that *APC* does not fulfil the role of a classic tumour suppressor as proposed by Knudson, in as much as the site of the germline mutation influences the site and type of 'second hit' in the wild-type *APC* allele (Lamlum *et al*. 1999).

APC is a large gene, but detection of mutation is simplified by the fact that about 90% of all mutations in FAP and sporadic adenomas occur within codons 1286–1513 of exon 15, known as the 'mutation cluster region' (MCR) (Miyoshi *et al*. 1992), and are truncating in nature. These facts are used to detect germline *APC* mutations in patients with a family history of FAP by the protein truncation test (PTT), an in vitro transcription–translation of the *APC* gene enabling the resolution of APC proteins on the basis of their molecular weight and, therefore, size (van der Luijt & van der Luijt 1996).

The nature of *APC* mutations and their clustering within a small region of the *APC* gene gives a clue as to the role of APC in polyp prevention. Although APC is a multifunctional protein, the most well elucidated of its roles is in forming a complex with the molecules axin and glycogen synthase kinase 3β, leading to binding and degradation of β-catenin (Hart *et al*. 1998; Ikeda *et al*. 1998; Itoh *et al*. 1998; Kishida *et al*. 1998; Sakanaka *et al*. 1998). Almost all mutations remove the SAMP (connexin/actin/β-catenin) repeats and all but one or two of the seven β-catenin-binding sites in *APC*, therefore preventing β-catenin degradation. In this situation, β-catenin can translocate to the nucleus and transcribe genes, such as c-*myc* (He *et al*. 1998), and cyclin D1 (Tetsu & McCormick 1999), which are associated with tumour cell growth and dysregulation of proliferation. This appears to be the fundamental mechanism by which most heritable and sporadic adenomas are initiated.

Some patients fulfilling criteria for FAP are found to have no mutation in the MCR (*APC* negative). There are two possible reasons for this: (1) there is a mutation outside the MCR; (2) there is no APC mutation. These latter cases may have mutations in other genes, leading to polyp development.

Genotype–phenotype correlations in FAP

The correlation between site of germline *APC* mutation and patient characteristics provides an excellent example of how knowledge of molecular biology can help to predict disease severity and presence of extraintestinal manifestations, and help to tailor treatment for tumours with specific mutations.

Although caused by a mutation in a single gene, with almost 100% penetrance, polyp burden and presence of extraintestinal manifestations vary widely both within and, particularly, between FAP kindreds. The most severe disease is associated with mutations around codon 1300 (Gayther *et al*. 1994), whereas mild disease is associated with truncating mutations in the 5′ (proximal) or 3′ (distal) regions of the *APC* gene (so-called attenuated FAP [AFAP]) (Spirio *et al*. 1993; Friedl *et al*. 1996). This seems to apply more to colorectal polyps than to upper gastrointestinal polyps. The reasons for these genotype–phenotype correlations are not completely understood, but may relate to stability of the different APC mutant proteins generated. Knowledge of these correlations allows one to predict which FAP patients may be at higher risk for early onset of cancer (i.e. high polyp count). Furthermore, a study from Leiden (Vasen *et al*. 1996b) has shown that it is reasonable clinical practice to leave the rectum *in situ* (i.e. perform an ileorectal anastomosis) in patients with APC mutations before codon 1250, whereas excision of the rectum should be undertaken in patients whose mutation occurs after this codon.

Presence of extraintestinal manifestations is also partially accounted for by site of germline mutation. Desmoid formation is associated with mutations between codons 1403 and 1578 (Caspari *et al*. 1995) and congenital hypertrophy of retinal pigmented epithelium (CHRPE) occurs only in patients with mutations between codons 463 and 1387 (Olschwang *et al*. 1993).

FAP: modifiers of phenotype

Although the site of the germline *APC* mutation in FAP has a large impact on disease severity, it does not completely account for differences between patients. Several modifier genes influencing polyp burden in the *min* (multiple intestinal neoplasia) mouse model of FAP have been identified. Such genes include phospholipase A$_2$, cyclo-oxygenase 2, DNA methylenetetrahydrofolate reductase and *Smad4* (Laird *et al*. 1995; MacPhee *et al*. 1995; Oshima *et al*. 1996; Takaku *et al*. 1998). Evidence for the existence of homologous human genes mediating similar effects in FAP have so far not been demonstrated, although it is likely that they may act as low-penetrance risk alleles in sporadic colorectal cancer also (Houlston & Tomlinson 1998). In addition, the colonic microenvironment is likely to influence the number of polyps formed, e.g. increased polyp number in patients with high levels of circulating carcinogens.

Hereditary non-polyposis colorectal cancer
Molecular basis of HNPCC

As with FAP, HNPCC is autosomally dominantly inherited (Lynch & Lynch 1985), but displays a penetrance of 80–85% for colon cancer and 40–45% for endometrial cancer (the major extracolonic manifestation) (Dunlop *et al*. 1997; Aarnio *et al*. 1999). As the name suggests, most colon tumours occurring in patients with HNPCC tend to occur without a recognisable precursor polyp.

The characteristic genotypic alteration seen in HNPCC tumours is microsatellite instability (MSI/MIN). These tumours are thus termed 'MSI+', and show random errors of replication (RER+), i.e. mutations in DNA microsatellites (Ionov *et al*. 1993; Shibata *et al*. 1994). Linkage studies in HNPCC kindreds led to the discovery of two mismatch repair (*MMR*) genes, termed '*hMLH1*' and '*hMSH2*'; mutations in these account for 45–86% of all classic HNPCC families (Fishel *et al*. 1993; Leach *et al*. 1993; Peltomaki *et al*. 1993; Bronner *et al*. 1994; Papadopoulos *et al*. 1994; Peltomaki & de la Chapelle 1997). Four other human MMR enzymes have subsequently been discovered. The mismatch repair system is highly conserved from bacteria through to higher organisms, and serves to detect and initiate repair of nucleotide base mispairing occurring during DNA replication (Harfe & Jinks-Robertson 2000). These enzymes have been termed 'caretakers' of the genome and mutation of these genes has been likened to constant exposure of the genome to a highly mutagenic environment (Kinzler & Vogelstein 1998). Patients with HNPCC display a particular mutational spectrum involving genes containing microsatellites, e.g. transforming growth factor β-II (TGF-βII) receptor, IGF-II receptor and Bax (Markowitz *et al*. 1995; Souza *et al*. 1996; Rampino *et al*. 1997), which are involved in cell growth and apoptosis control.

Microsatellite instability also occurs in sporadic colorectal cancer. It is a general principle that, whereas in HNPCC *MMR* genes are mutated, in sporadic tumours showing MSI there is epigenetic inactivation of *MMR* genes, usually involving promoter methylation (Kane *et al*. 1997; Herman *et al*. 1998; Cunningham *et al*. 1998; Veigl *et al*. 1998; Wheeler *et al*. 1999). Indeed, MMR enzymes may act as true tumour-suppressor genes, in that somatic loss of the wild-type allele is often seen in HNPCC tumours (Hemminki *et al*. 1994).

Of all patients fulfilling the Amsterdam criteria (see Chapter 3, page 39) for a diagnosis of HNPCC, 10–40% do not have a recognised mutation in an MMR enzyme. This may be the result of inability to detect the mutation, or of a germline mutation in a gene typically mutated in HNPCC tumours, giving a similar phenotype, e.g. TGF-βII receptor (Lu *et al.* 1998).

Genotype–phenotype correlations in HNPCC

The precise molecular defect in an HNPCC patient can help to predict the phenotype, e.g. *hMSH2* mutation carriers have a higher incidence of extracolonic neoplasms than those with *hMLH1* mutations (Vasen *et al.* 1996b). Similarly, patients with a germline mutation in *hMSH6* develop endometrial cancer at a higher rate than colon cancer (Wijnen *et al.* 1999). These facts are obviously extremely important in designing screening regimens for extracolonic neoplasms in these patients.

There is some evidence that phenotypic variability between HNPCC patients with the same germline mutation may be the result of modifier factors. The *N*-acetyl-transferase 1 (NAT1) polymorphism is associated with early age of colon cancer onset in HNPCC patients (Moisio *et al.* 1998). NAT is involved in carcinogen metabolism, providing an example of interaction between genetic and environmental factors in tumour development.

Peutz–Jeghers syndrome

Peutz–Jeghers syndrome is characterised by the development of numerous hamartomatous polyps within the gastrointestinal tract, and is inherited in an autosomal dominant fashion. It is uncertain whether the hamartomas represent a preneoplastic lesion, but gastrointestinal cancers are more common in these patients than in the general population (Giardiello *et al.* 2000). Loss of heterozygosity of the *LKB1* and *Smad4* genes have been implicated in the genesis of the Peutz–Jeghers syndrome (Hemminki *et al.* 1998; Howe *et al.* 1998; Jenne *et al.* 1998; Miyaki *et al.* 2000; Woodford-Richens *et al.* 2000). It appears, furthermore, that both of these genes may act as tumour suppressors, with mutation of one allele inherited in the germline, and a 'second hit' mutation of the wild-type allele occurring during polyp formation.

Hyperplastic polyposis syndrome

Hyperplastic polyposis syndrome (HPS) is characterised by multiple, often large, hyperplastic polyps located throughout the large bowel. In contradistinction from sporadic hyperplastic polyps, HPS polyps often display atypical cytological features (Williams *et al.* 1980; Jeevaratnam *et al.* 1996; Torlakovic & Snover 1996). The molecular characteristics of HPS are only just beginning to be elucidated, and it is unsure whether carcinomatous change occurs within these lesions through a hyperplasia–adenoma–carcinoma sequence. Conflicting reports suggest that carcinoma arising in a patient with HPS occurs by a predominantly CIN (Hawkins *et al.* 2000; Rashid *et al.* 2000) or MIN (Iino *et al.* 1999, 2000; Jass *et al.* 2000) pathway. In reality it is likely that, as with most sporadic colorectal cancers, elements of both CIN and MIN are present in these tumours. The predominant importance of one element over the other is difficult to ascertain when taking a 'snapshot' of the molecular changes present in a tumour at any point in time. Moreover, it is likely that both elements co-operate in the initiation and development of a tumour.

The adenoma–carcinoma sequence

Background

The evolution of colorectal cancer from adenomas, first described by Morson (1974), is accepted as the manner by which most tumours arise. The progression of adenoma to carcinoma involves epigenetic events, mutations, over-expression and losses of several key genes, often at particular stages of tumour evolution, as originally proposed by Fearon and Vogelstein (1990). There is, however, considerable heterogeneity in the mutational spectrum between individual tumours, and it is recognised that the chronological order of mutation acquisition is not as important as the overall number and type of mutations gained.

Molecular events

Figure 2.1 shows common mutational events and frequent stage of occurrence during the adenoma–carcinoma sequence. Molecular and clinical correlates for genes implicated in the adenoma–carcinoma sequence are discussed below.

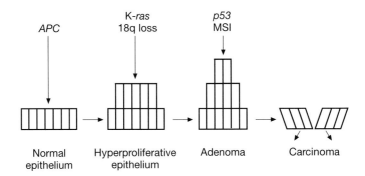

Figure 2.1 Adenoma–carcinoma sequence.

Adenomatous polyposis coli

As has been stated in the context of FAP, *APC* truncation is the most common early event in adenoma formation, and at least 63% of early adenomas will contain an *APC* truncation in the MCR alone (Powell *et al*. 1992). Indeed, it has been shown that *APC* mutation alone is sufficient for the growth of most adenomas up to 1 cm (Lamlum *et al*. 2000). *APC* mutation is thought to allow epithelial hyperproliferation, an early stage in adenoma initiation. Around 50% of adenomas that do not have an *APC* mutation have an activating mutation of β-catenin (Sparks *et al.* 1998), and it appears that these two mutations can to some extent compensate for one another. This fact can be rationalised when it is remembered that a major function of *APC* is to degrade β-catenin. Of the adenomas without either an *APC* or a β-catenin mutation, some will be found to be MSI+; however, MSI more usually occurs during the later stages of the adenoma–carcinoma sequence.

K-ras

Mutation in the oncogene K-*ras* occurs at an intermediate–late stage in adenoma progression, at frequencies of 40–70%. K-*ras* operates as a molecular switch in several signal transduction pathways controlling cell proliferation, differentiation and apoptosis (Lowy & Willumsen 1993). K-*ras* mutations in colorectal cancer constitutively activate K-*ras*, leading to continual activation of *ras* signalling pathways. The incidence of K-*ras* mutation increases with increased adenoma size and degree of dysplasia (Vogelstein *et al.* 1988; McLellan *et al.* 1993). The molecular nature of the K-*ras* mutation influences the malignant potential of tumour cells:

- K-*ras* codon 12 mutations are more common in carcinomas than in adenomas (Capella *et al.* 1991), and metastatic compared with non-metastatic lesions (Finkelstein *et al.* 1993a, 1993b).
- K-*ras* codon 13 mutations are found exclusively in tumours that show no local invasion (Finkelstein *et al.* 1993a).
- K-*ras* codon 12 mutation induces higher levels of apoptosis resistance and predisposition to anchorage-independent growth than codon 13 mutations (Guerrero *et al.* 2000).

These studies suggest that codon 12 mutations lead to a more aggressive phenotype than codon 13 mutations.

Chromosome 18q

Losses of chromosome 18q occur in 60–80% of late adenomas. Three putative tumour-suppressor genes have been studied on chromosome 18q: deleted in colon cancer (*DCC*) (Fearon & Vogelstein 1990; Fearon *et al.* 1990), *Smad2* (Eppert *et al.* 1996; Riggins *et al.* 1996) and *Smad4* (Hahn *et al.* 1996).

   DCC encodes for a transmembrane protein that may function as a receptor for the axonal chemoattractant nettrin-1 (Keino-Masu *et al.* 1996). The main contentious issue regarding a role for *DCC* in colorectal cancer formation is whether expression of the *DCC* gene product is decreased in adenoma–carcinoma progression, with conflicting results in studies to date (Cho *et al.* 1994; Shibata *et al.* 1996; Fazeli *et al.* 1997; Chen *et al.* 1999; Fabre *et al.* 1999).

Smad2 and *Smad4* genes encode proteins that play an essential role in TGF-β signalling pathways. Under normal conditions, TGF-β is a potent anti-mitogen in epithelial cells (Massagué *et al.* 1990) and loss of TGF-β antiproliferative responses in colon carcinoma cells may favour tumour formation. This loss of responsiveness can result from inactivating mutations in TGF-β receptor genes, particularly in the context of microsatellite instability, or mutation/inactivation of other components of the TGF-β signalling pathway (i.e. *Smad2*, *Smad4*). *Smad2* gene mutations have been identified in a small proportion of colorectal cancers (Eppert *et al.* 1996) and *Smad4* is structurally altered in a significant proportion of colorectal carcinomas (Takagi *et al.* 1996; Thiagalingam *et al.* 1996; Hoque *et al.* 1997; MacGrogan *et al.* 1997).

Allelic losses of chromosome 18q may predict a poor outcome in patients with colorectal cancer (Jen *et al.* 1994; Martínez-López *et al.* 1998), and in particular *Smad4* dysfunction has been associated with metastatic potential (Miyaki *et al.* 1999). The increased susceptibility to colorectal cancer observed in *Smad4/min* mice mutants has further implicated this gene in colorectal tumorigenesis (Takaku *et al.* 1998).

It is not entirely certain what proportion of *DCC*, *Smad2* and *Smad4* loci are inactivated in particular colorectal tumours, but attempts to answer this question using the technique of xenografting of colorectal tumours into mice has suggested that *Smad4* was the deletion target in a third of the tumours, and that DCC or a neighbouring gene was the target in the remaining two-thirds (Thiagalingam *et al.* 1996).

p53

The p53 protein is also known as the 'guardian of the genome', a reference to its properties as a central regulator of the cell cycle. It is a phosphoprotein nuclear transcription factor (Farmer *et al.* 1992; Kern *et al.* 1992) which oligomerises and binds to DNA-recognition sequences adjacent to *p53*-responsive genes, inducing cell cycle arrest (el-Deiry *et al.* 1993) and apoptosis (Miyashita & Reed 1995) in cells with damaged DNA, thus preventing proliferation and division of such cells.

Around 75% of late colorectal adenomas and carcinomas contain mutations in the *p53* gene, most commonly missense point mutations clustered in the central, DNA-binding domain (Hollstein *et al.* 1991; Cho *et al.* 1994). The mutant proteins thus formed are incapable of binding to DNA and regulating expression of *p53*-responsive genes (Kern *et al.* 1991, 1992; el-Deiry *et al.* 1992, 1993; Farmer *et al.* 1992; Cho *et al.* 1994; Miyashita & Reed 1995). A further mechanism by which some *p53* mutations can interfere with cell cycle regulation is by the binding and inactivation of wild-type p53 protein (Milner & Medcalf 1991; Harvey *et al.* 1995).

Wild-type p53 protein is not detectable in normal cell nuclei; however, mutant protein shows increased stability and nuclear accumulation. Immunohistochemical nuclear p53 staining therefore implies mutant protein in most cases. As with many other alterations, p53 has been studied as a possible molecular marker for adenoma recurrence, metastasis and survival in colorectal cancer, often with conflicting results (Triantafyllou *et al.* 1999; Bouzourene *et al.* 2000; Gallego *et al.* 2000; Kahlenberg *et al.* 2000; Makino *et al.* 2000). It appears that mutant p53 expression may be an independent negative prognostic factor, but the data are perhaps not rigorous enough at present to recommend use of this molecular marker in routine clinical practice.

Cyclo-oxygenase 2

Cyclo-oxygenase 2 (COX-2) is an inducible enzyme stimulated by inflammatory mediators which may play a role in wound healing within the gastrointestinal tract (Sakamoto 1998). Several studies have implicated COX-2 over-expression in the pathogenesis of the adenoma–carcinoma sequence (Eberhart *et al.* 1994; Sano *et al.* 1995; Williams *et al.* 1996), although the mechanism by which such over-expression may influence tumorigenesis is so far largely unclear. Therapeutic trials of COX-2 inhibitors in patients with FAP and *min* mice have yielded encouraging results in the prevention and regression of adenomas and cancers (Kune *et al.* 1988; Thun *et al.* 1991; Giardiello *et al.* 1993; Jacoby *et al.* 1996; Oshima *et al.* 1996), suggesting that these agents will become a useful therapeutic intervention in the prevention of colorectal cancer.

Other implicated loci and genes

Many other genetic loci and gene products have been implicated in the adenoma–carcinoma sequence, and there is insufficient space here to detail the available evidence. Such loci include 1p, 3p, 8p, 9p, 13q, 16q, 22q and HLA. Proteins thought to be involved in colorectal tumorigenesis include bax, bcl-2, p16, p21, cyclin D1, cyclin-dependent kinases, fez-1, retinoblastoma protein, telomerase and von Hippel–Landau protein.

Ulcerative colitis-associated colorectal cancer

Background

Chronic (>8 years' duration), extensive ulcerative colitis is associated with a two- to eightfold increased risk of colorectal cancer over non-colitic populations. Cancer in ulcerative colitis is thought to arise through a number of sequential precursor lesions, namely indeterminate, low-grade and high-grade dysplasia. The inclusion of indeterminate dysplasia in the sequence underlines a major difficulty in this area – assessing the significance of indeterminate or mild dysplastic change. Three problems account for this difficulty:

1. Sampling error: dysplastic change is often patchy and there are no macroscopically visible indicators of dysplasia in ulcerative colitis to guide biopsy.
2. The uncertainty whether mild dysplastic change is associated with an increased cancer risk.

3. Intra- and interobserver variation in diagnosis of dysplasia, even among experienced gastrointestinal pathologists.

Non-dysplastic mucosa from chronic ulcerative colitis has been found to show microsatellite instability (Brentnall *et al.* 1996), chromosomal instability (Willenbucher *et al.* 1997; Rabinovitch *et al.* 1999) and *p53* mutations (Hussain *et al.* 2000). One interpretation of these studies is that molecular changes occur in ulcerative colitis mucosa before histologically identifiable dysplasia. Whether such molecular markers imply an increased predisposition to cancer development is uncertain, as is their potential use as screening markers in combination with histological criteria.

Molecular changes in ulcerative colitis dysplasia and carcinoma

Many molecular alterations occurring in the ulcerative colitis–dysplasia–carcinoma sequence are similar in nature to those occurring in the adenoma–carcinoma sequence. The major differences between these two pathways appears to be in timing and rate of specific genetic alterations. Table 2.2 compares and contrasts these two sequences. The rates of alterations given in Table 2.2 are imprecise – because of the difficulty in diagnosing dysplasia in ulcerative colitis, studies often give conflicting results. In particular, the importance of MSI (Cawkwell *et al.* 2000; Fleischer *et al.* 2000; Lyda *et al.* 2000) and especially the possible role of *MSH2* germline mutation (Brentnall *et al.* 1995; Noffsinger *et al.* 1999) in dysplasia and cancer development in ulcerative colitis appears uncertain. The most apparent molecular difference between the two sequences is the low rate of *APC* mutation in ulcerative colitis dysplasia versus sporadic adenomas (Tarmin *et al.* 1995). As has been discussed, *APC* mutation is thought to lead to increased proliferation in colonic mucosa. In the context of ulcerative colitis, the balance between cell proliferation and death is already disturbed, and *APC* mutation does not appear to be a necessary initial transforming step.

Table 2.2 Comparison of molecular events and their timing in the adenoma–carcinoma (AC) and ulcerative colitis–dysplasia–carcinoma (UCDC) sequences

	AC	UCDC
p53 mutation	Late, ~75%	Early, ~90%
APC mutation	Early, ~70%	Late, ~6%
K-*ras* mutation	~50%	~30%
Microsatellite instability	Late, 10–15%	Early, ~20%
18q loss	Intermediate, ~80%	Early, 75%

Dysplasia-associated lesion or mass

The differentiation of simple adenoma from dysplasia-associated lesion or mass (DALM) is very difficult histologically, but has huge management implications – the choice of simple polypectomy for adenoma or colectomy for DALM, given the high incidence of related cancer. An attempt has been made to identify molecular markers that can differentiate between these two lesions (Fogt *et al.* 1998; Walsh *et al.* 1999; Odze *et al.* 2000), the results of which are presented in Table 2.3. The combination of such molecular analysis, combined with standard clinicopathological variables shows promise in this difficult area.

Table 2.3 Comparison of molecular features of sporadic adenoma arising in chronic ulcerative colitis and dysplasia-associated lesion or mass (DALM)

	Sporadic adenoma	*DALM*
p53 staining	Weak or absent	Strong, diffuse
β-Catenin staining	Strong, diffuse	Weak or absent
LOH for VHL	Uncommon	Common
LOH for p16	Rare	Common
LOH for p53	Rare	Common

LOH, loss of heterozygosity; VHL, von Hippel–Landau.

Conclusions

Understanding of the molecular biology of colorectal cancer is progressing at a rapid rate. At present the major applications of this knowledge to the clinical field of colorectal cancer management are in the diagnosis, screening and rational therapeutic intervention of patients with genetic syndromes that have a predisposition to colorectal cancer. In addition, promise is being shown in using molecular markers as prognostic indicators and diagnostic aids. It is likely that future developments in cancer genome screening and tumour molecular profiling will rapidly expand the use of molecular tools in routine clinical practice.

References

Aarnio M, Sankila R, Pukkala E *et al.* (1999). Cancer risk in mutation carriers of DNA-mismatch-repair genes. *International Journal of Cancer* **81**, 214–218

Bale SJ, Chakravarti A, Strong LC (1984). Aggregation of colon cancer in family data. *Genetic Epidemiology* **1**(1): 53–61

Baylin SB, Hoppener JW, de Bustres A *et al.* (1986). DNA methylation patterns of the calcitonin gene in human lung cancers and lymphomas. *Cancer Research* **46**, 2917–2922

Bodmer WF, Bailey CJ, Bodmer J *et al.* (1987). Localization of the gene for familial adenomatous polyposis on chromosome 5. *Nature* **328**, 614–616

Bouzourene H, Gervaz P, Cerottini JP *et al.* (2000). p53 and Ki-*ras* as prognostic factors for Dukes stage B colorectal cancer. *European Journal of Cancer* **36**, 1008–1015

Brentnall, TA, Rubin CE, Crispin DA *et al*. (1995). A germline substitution in the human MSH2 gene is associated with high-grade dysplasia and cancer in ulcerative colitis [see comments]. *Gastroenterology* **109**, 151–155

Brentnall TA, Crispin DA, Bronner MP *et al*. (1996). Microsatellite instability in nonneoplastic mucosa from patients with chronic ulcerative colitis. *Cancer Research* **56**, 1237–1240

Bronner CE, Baker SM, Morrison PT *et al*. (1994). Mutation in the DNA mismatch repair gene homologue hMLH1 is associated with hereditary non-polyposis colon cancer. *Nature* **368**, 258–61

Burt RW, Bishop DT, Cannon LA, Doudle MA, Lee RG, Skolnick MH (1985). Dominant inheritance of adenomatous colonic polyps and colorectal cancer. *New England Journal of Medicine* **312**, 1540–1544

Capella G, Cronauer-Mitra S, Pienado MA *et al*. (1991). Frequency and spectrum of mutations at codons 12 and 13 of the c-K-*ras* gene in human tumors. *Environmental Health Perspective* **93**, 125–131

Carstensen B, Soll-Johanning H, Villadsen E *et al*. (1996). Familial aggregation of colorectal cancer in the general population. *International Journal of Cancer* **68**, 428–435

Caspari R, Olschwang S, Friedl W *et al*. (1995). Familial adenomatous polyposis: desmoid tumours and lack of ophthalmic lesions (CHRPE) associated with APC mutations beyond codon 1444. *Human Molecular Genetics* **4**, 337–340

Cawkwell L, Sutherland F, Murgatroyd H *et al*. (2000). Defective hMSH2/hMLH1 protein expression is seen infrequently in ulcerative colitis associated colorectal cancers [see comments]. *Gut* **46**, 367–369

Chen YQ, Hsieh JT, Yao F *et al*. (1999). Induction of apoptosis and G2/M cell cycle arrest by DCC. *Oncogene* **18**, 2747–2754

Cho KR, Oliner JD, Simons JW *et al*. (1994). The DCC gene: structural analysis and mutations in colorectal carcinomas. *Genomics* **19**, 525–531

Cui H, Horon IL, Ohlsson R *et al*. (1998). Loss of imprinting in normal tissue of colorectal cancer patients with microsatellite instability [see comments]. *Nature Medicine* **4**, 1276–1280

Cunningham JM, Christensen ER, Tester DJ *et al*. (1998). Hypermethylation of the hMLH1 promoter in colon cancer with microsatellite instability. *Cancer Research* **58**, 3455–3460

Dunlop MG, Farrington SM, Carothers AD *et al*. (1997). Cancer risk associated with germline DNA mismatch repair gene mutations. *Human Molecular Genetics* **6**, 105–110

Eberhart CE, Coffey RJ, Radhika A *et al*. (1994). Up-regulation of cyclooxygenase 2 gene expression in human colorectal adenomas and adenocarcinomas. *Gastroenterology* **107**, 1183–1188

el-Deiry WS, Kern SE, Pietenpol JA *et al*. (1992). Definition of a consensus binding site for p53. *Nature Genetics* **1**, 45–49

el-Deiry WS, Tokino T, Velculescu VE *et al*. (1993). WAF1, a potential mediator of p53 tumor suppression. *Cell* **75**, 817–825

Eppert K, Scherer SW, Ozcelik H *et al*. (1996). MADR2 maps to 18q21 and encodes a TGFbeta-regulated MAD-related protein that is functionally mutated in colorectal carcinoma. *Cell* **86**, 543–552

Fabre M, Martin M, Ulloa F *et al*. (1999). In vitro analysis of the role of DCC in mucus-secreting intestinal differentiation. *International Journal of Cancer* **81**, 799–807

Farmer G, Bargonetti J, Zhu H *et al*. (1992). Wild-type p53 activates transcription in vitro [see comments]. *Nature* **358**, 83–86

Fazeli A, Dickinson SL, Hermiston ML *et al*. (1997). Phenotype of mice lacking functional Deleted in colorectal cancer (Dcc) gene. *Nature* **386**, 796–804

Fearon ER & Vogelstein B (1990). A genetic model for colorectal tumorigenesis. *Cell* **61**, 759–767

Fearon ER, Cho KR, Nigro JM *et al.* (1990). Identification of a chromosome 18q gene that is altered in colorectal cancers. *Science* **247**, 49–56

Feinberg AP & Vogelstein B (1983). Hypomethylation distinguishes genes of some human cancers from their normal counterparts. *Nature* **301**, 89–92

Feinberg AP, Gehrke CW, Kvo KC *et al.* (1988). Reduced genomic 5-methylcytosine content in human colonic neoplasia. *Cancer Research* **48**, 1159–1161

Finkelstein SD, Sayegh R, Christenson S *et al.* (1993a). Determination of tumor aggressiveness in colorectal cancer by K-*ras*-2 analysis. *Archives of Surgery* **128**, 526–531; discussion 531–532

Finkelstein SD, Sayegh R, Bakker A *et al.* (1993b). Genotypic classification of colorectal adenocarcinoma. Biologic behavior correlates with K-*ras*-2 mutation type. *Cancer* **71**, 3827–3838

Fishel R, Lescoe MK, Rao MR *et al.* (1993). The human mutator gene homolog MSH2 and its association with hereditary nonpolyposis colon cancer [published erratum appears in *Cell* 1994 April 8; **77**, 167]. *Cell* **75**, 1027–1038

Fleisher AS, Esteller M, Harpaz N *et al.* (2000). Microsatellite instability in inflammatory bowel disease-associated neoplastic lesions is associated with hypermethylation and diminished expression of the DNA mismatch repair gene, hMLH1. *Cancer Research* **60**, 4864–4868

Fogt F, Vortmeyer AO, Stolte M *et al.* (1998). Loss of heterozygosity of the von Hippel Lindau gene locus in polypoid dysplasia but not flat dysplasia in ulcerative colitis or sporadic adenomas. *Human Pathology* **29**, 961–964

Friedl W, Meuschel S, Caspari R *et al.* (1996). Attenuated familial adenomatous polyposis due to a mutation in the 3 part of the APC gene. A clue for understanding the function of the APC protein. *Human Genetics* **97**, 579–584

Gallego MG, Acenero MJ, Ortega S *et al.* (2000). Prognostic influence of p53 nuclear overexpression in colorectal carcinoma. *Diseases of the Colon and Rectum* **43**, 971–975

Gayther SA, Wells D, Sen Gupta SB *et al.* (1994). Regionally clustered APC mutations are associated with a severe phenotype and occur at a high frequency in new mutation cases of adenomatous polyposis coli. *Human Molecular Genetics* **3**, 53–56

Georgiades IB, Curtis LJ, Morris RM *et al.* (1999). Heterogeneity studies identify a subset of sporadic colorectal cancers without evidence for chromosomal or microsatellite instability. *Oncogene* **18**, 7933–4790

Giardiello FM, Hamilton SR, Krush AJ *et al.* (1993). Treatment of colonic and rectal adenomas with sulindac in familial adenomatous polyposis. *New England Journal of Medicine* **328**, 1313–1316

Giardiello FM, Brensinger JD, Tersmette AC *et al.* (2000). Very high risk of cancer in familial Peutz–Jeghers syndrome [In Process Citation]. *Gastroenterology* **119**, 1447–1453

Guerrero S, Casanova I, Farre L *et al.* (2000). K-ras codon 12 mutation induces higher level of resistance to apoptosis and predisposition to anchorage-independent growth than codon 13 mutation or proto-oncogene overexpression [In Process Citation]. *Cancer Research* **60**, 6750–6756

Hahn SA, Schutte M, Hoque AT *et al.* (1996). DPC4, a candidate tumor suppressor gene at human chromosome 18q21.1. [see comments]. *Science* **271**, 350–353

Hardy RG, Meltzer SJ, Jankowski JA *et al.* (2001). ABC of colorectal cancer. Molecular basis for risk factors. *British Medical Journal* **321**, 886

Harfe BD & Jinks-Robertson S (2000). DNA mismatch repair and genetic instability. *Annual Review of Genetics* **3**, 359–399

Hart MJ, de los Santos R, Albert IN *et al*. (1998). Downregulation of β-catenin by human Axin and its association with the APC tumor suppressor, β-catenin and GSK3 β. *Current Biology* **8**, 573–581

Harvey M, Vogel H, Morris D *et al*. (1995). A mutant p53 transgene accelerates tumour development in heterozygous but not nullizygous p53-deficient mice. *Nature Genetics* **9**, 305–311

Hawkins NJ, Gorman P, Tomlinson IP *et al*. (2000). Colorectal carcinomas arising in the hyperplastic polyposis syndrome progress through the chromosomal instability pathway. *American Journal of Pathology* **157**, 385–392

He TC, Sparks AB, Rago C *et al*. (1998). Identification of c-MYC as a target of the APC pathway [see comments]. *Science* **281**, 1509–1512

Hemminki A, Peltomaki P, Mecklin JP *et al*. (1994). Loss of the wild type MLH1 gene is a feature of hereditary nonpolyposis colorectal cancer. *Nature Genetics* **8**, 405–410

Hemminki A, Markie D, Tomlinson I *et al*. (1998). A serine/threonine kinase gene defective in Peutz–Jeghers syndrome. *Nature* **391**, 184–187

Herman JG, Umar A, Polyak K *et al*. (1998). Incidence and functional consequences of hMLH1 promoter hypermethylation in colorectal carcinoma. *Proceedings of the National Academy of Sciences of the USA* **95**, 6870–6875

Hollstein M, Sidransky D, Vogelstein B *et al*. (1991). p53 mutations in human cancers. *Science* **253**, 49–53

Hoque AT, Hahn SA, Schutte M *et al*. (1997). DPC4 gene mutation in colitis associated neoplasia. *Gut* **40**, 120–122

Houlston RS & Tomlinson IP (1998). Modifier genes in humans: strategies for identification. *European Journal of Human Genetics* **6**, 80–88

Howe JR, Roth S, Ringold JC *et al*. (1998). Mutations in the SMAD4/DPC4 gene in juvenile polyposis [see comments]. *Science* **280**, 1086–1088

Hussain SP, Amstad P, Raja K *et al*. (2000). Increased p53 mutation load in noncancerous colon tissue from ulcerative colitis: a cancer-prone chronic inflammatory disease. *Cancer Research* **60**, 3333–3337

Iino H, Jass JR, Simms LA *et al*. (1999). DNA microsatellite instability in hyperplastic polyps, serrated adenomas, and mixed polyps: a mild mutator pathway for colorectal cancer? *Journal of Clinical Pathology* **52**, 5–9

Iino H, Simms L, Young J *et al*. (2000). DNA microsatellite instability and mismatch repair protein loss in adenomas presenting in hereditary non-polyposis colorectal cancer. *Gut* **47**, 37–42

Ikeda S, Kishida S, Yamamoto H *et al*. (1998). Axin, a negative regulator of the Wnt signaling pathway, forms a complex with GSK-3β and β-catenin and promotes GSK-3β-dependent phosphorylation of β-catenin. *EMBO Journal* **17**, 1371–1384

Ionov Y, Peinado MA, Malkhosyun S *et al*. (1993). Ubiquitous somatic mutations in simple repeated sequences reveal a new mechanism for colonic carcinogenesis. *Nature* **363**, 558–561

Itoh K, Krupnik VE, Sokol SY *et al*. (1998). Axis determination in *Xenopus* involves biochemical interactions of axin, glycogen synthase kinase 3 and β-catenin. *Current Biology* **8**, 591–594

Jacoby RF, Marshall DJ, Newton MA *et al*. (1996). Chemoprevention of spontaneous intestinal adenomas in the Apc Min mouse model by the nonsteroidal anti-inflammatory drug piroxicam. *Cancer Research* **56**, 710–714

Jass JR, Iino H, Ruszkiewicz A *et al*. (2000). Neoplastic progression occurs through mutator pathways in hyperplastic polyposis of the colorectum. *Gut* **47**, 43–49

Jeevaratnam P, Cottier DS, Browett PS *et al*. (1996). Familial giant hyperplastic polyposis predisposing to colorectal cancer: a new hereditary bowel cancer syndrome. *Journal of Pathology* **179**, 20–25

Jen J, Kim H, Piantadosi S *et al*. (1994). Allelic loss of chromosome 18q and prognosis in colorectal cancer [see comments]. *New England Journal of Medicine* **331**, 213–221

Jenne DE, Reimann H, Nezu J *et al*. (1998). Peutz–Jeghers syndrome is caused by mutations in a novel serine threonine kinase. *Nature Genetics* **18**, 38–43

Kahlenberg MS, Stoler DL, Rodriguez-Biggs M *et al*. (2000). p53 tumor suppressor gene mutations predict decreased survival of patients with sporadic colorectal carcinoma. *Cancer* **88**, 1814–1819

Kane MF, Loda M, Gaida GM *et al*. (1997). Methylation of the hMLH1 promoter correlates with lack of expression of hMLH1 in sporadic colon tumors and mismatch repair-defective human tumor cell lines. *Cancer Research* **57**, 808–811

Keino-Masu K, Masu M, Hinck L *et al*. (1996). Deleted in colorectal cancer (DCC) encodes a netrin receptor. *Cell* **87**, 175–185

Kern SE, Kinzler KW, Baker SJ *et al*. (1991). Mutant p53 proteins bind DNA abnormally in vitro. *Oncogene* **6**, 131–136

Kern SE, Pietenpol JA, Thiagalingam S *et al*. (1992). Oncogenic forms of p53 inhibit p53-regulated gene expression. *Science* **256**, 827–830

Kinzler KW & Vogelstein B (1996). Lessons from hereditary colorectal cancer. *Cell* **87**, 159–170

Kinzler KW & Vogelstein B (1998). Landscaping the cancer terrain [comment]. *Science* **280**, 1036–1037

Kishida S, Yamamoto H, Ikeda S *et al*. (1998). Axin, a negative regulator of the wnt signaling pathway, directly interacts with adenomatous polyposis coli and regulates the stabilization of β-catenin. *Journal of Biological Chemistry* **273**, 10823–10826

Kune GA, Kune S, Watson LF (1988). Colorectal cancer risk, chronic illnesses, operations, and medications: case control results from the Melbourne Colorectal Cancer Study. *Cancer Research* **48**, 4399–404

Laird PW, Jackson-Grusby L, Fazeli A *et al*. (1995). Suppression of intestinal neoplasia by DNA hypomethylation. *Cell* **81**, 197–205

Lamlum H, Ilyas M, Rowan A *et al*. (1999). The type of somatic mutation at APC in familial adenomatous polyposis is determined by the site of the germline mutation: a new facet to Knudson's two-hit hypothesis. *Nature Medicine* **5**, 1071–1075

Lamlum H, Papadopoulou A, Ilyas M *et al*. (2000). APC mutations are sufficient for the growth of early colorectal adenomas. *Proceedings of the National Academy of Sciences of the USA* **97**, 2225–2228

Leach FS, Nicolaides NC, Papadopoulos N *et al*. (1993). Mutations of a mutS homolog in hereditary nonpolyposis colorectal cancer. *Cell* **75**, 1215–1225

Lengauer C, Kinzler KW, Vogelstein B *et al*. (1998). Genetic instabilities in human cancers. *Nature* **396**, 643–649

Leppert M, Dobbs M, Scambler P *et al*. (1987). The gene for familial polyposis coli maps to the long arm of chromosome 5. *Science* **238**, 1411–1413

Lovett E (1976). Family studies in cancer of the colon and rectum. *British Journal of Surgery* **63**, 13–18

Lowy DR & Willumsen BM (1993). Function and regulation of *ras*. *Annual Review of Biochemistry* **62**, 851–891

Lu SL, Kawabata M, Imamura T *et al.* (1998). HNPCC associated with germline mutation in the TGF-β type II receptor gene [letter]. *Nature Genetics* **19**, 17–18

Lyda MH, Noffsinger A, Belli J *et al.* (2000). Microsatellite instability and K-*ras* mutations in patients with ulcerative colitis. *Human Pathology* **31**, 665–71

Lynch P & Lynch HT (1985). *Colon Cancer Genetics*. New York: Van Nostrand Rheinhold

MacGrogan D, Pegram M, Slamon D *et al.* (1997). Comparative mutational analysis of DPC4 (Smad4) in prostatic and colorectal carcinomas. *Oncogene* **15**, 1111–1114

McLellan EA, Owen RA, Stepniewska KA *et al.* (1993). High frequency of K-*ras* mutations in sporadic colorectal adenomas. *Gut* **34**, 392–396

MacPhee M, Chepenik KP, Liddell RA *et al.* (1995). The secretory phospholipase A2 gene is a candidate for the Mom1 locus, a major modifier of ApcMin-induced intestinal neoplasia. *Cell* **81**, 957–966

Makino M, Yamane N, Taniguchi T *et al.* (2000). p53 as an indicator of lymph node metastases in invasive early colorectal cancer. *Anticancer Research* **20**(3B), 2055–2059

Markowitz S, Wang J, Myeroff L *et al.* (1995). Inactivation of the type II TGF-β receptor in colon cancer cells with microsatellite instability [see comments]. *Science* **268**, 1336–1338

Martinez-Lopez E, Abad A, Font A *et al.* (1998). Allelic loss on chromosome 18q as a prognostic marker in stage II colorectal cancer [see comments]. *Gastroenterology* **114**, 1180–1187

Massagué J, Cheifetz S, Boyd FT *et al.* (1990). TGF-β receptors and TGF-β binding proteoglycans: recent progress in identifying their functional properties. *Annals of the New York Academy of Science* **593**, 59–72

Milner J & Medcalf EA (1991). Cotranslation of activated mutant p53 with wild type drives the wild-type p53 protein into the mutant conformation. *Cell* **65**, 765–774

Miyaki M, Iijima T, Konishi M *et al.* (1999). Higher frequency of Smad4 gene mutation in human colorectal cancer with distant metastasis. *Oncogene* **18**, 3098–3103

Miyaki M, Iijima T, Hosono K *et al.* (2000). Somatic mutations of LKB1 and β-catenin genes in gastrointestinal polyps from patients with Peutz-Jeghers syndrome [In Process Citation]. *Cancer Research* **60**, 6311–6313

Miyashita T & Reed JC (1995). Tumor suppressor p53 is a direct transcriptional activator of the human bax gene. *Cell* **80**, 293–209

Miyoshi Y, Nagase H, Ando H *et al.* (1992). Somatic mutations of the APC gene in colorectal tumors: mutation cluster region in the APC gene. *Human Molecular Genetics* **1**, 229–233

Moisio AL, Sistonen P, Mecklin JP *et al.* (1998). Genetic polymorphisms in carcinogen metabolism and their association to hereditary nonpolyposis colon cancer. *Gastroenterology* **115**, 1387–1394

Morson B (1974). Presidents address. The polyp-cancer sequence in the large bowel. *Proceedings of the Royal Society of Medicine* **67**, 451–457

Nakagawa H, Chadwick RB, Peltomaki P *et al.* (2001). Loss of imprinting of the insulin-like growth factor II gene occurs by biallelic methylation in a core region of H19-associated CTCF-binding sites in colorectal cancer. *Proceedings of the National Academy of Sciences of the USA* **98**, 591–596

Noffsinger AE, Belli JM, Fogt F (1999). A germline hMSH2 alteration is unrelated to colonic microsatellite instability in patients with ulcerative colitis. *Human Pathology* **30**, 8–12

Odze RD, Brown CA, Hartmann CJ *et al.* (2000). Genetic alterations in chronic ulcerative colitis-associated adenoma-like DALMs are similar to non-colitic sporadic adenomas. *American Journal of Surgical Pathology* **24**, 1209–1216

Olschwang S, Tiret A, Laurent-Puig P *et al.* (1993). Restriction of ocular fundus lesions to a specific subgroup of APC mutations in adenomatous polyposis coli patients. *Cell* **75**, 959–968

Oshima M, Dinchuk JE, Kargman SL *et al.* (1996). Suppression of intestinal polyposis in Apc delta716 knockout mice by inhibition of cyclooxygenase 2 (COX-2). *Cell* **87**, 803–809

Papadopoulos N, Nicolaides NC, Wei YF *et al.* (1994). Mutation of a mutL homolog in hereditary colon cancer [see comments]. *Science* **263**, 1625–1629

Peltomaki P, Aaltonen LA, Sistonen P *et al.* (1993). Genetic mapping of a locus predisposing to human colorectal cancer [see comments]. *Science* **260**, 810–812

Peltomaki P & de la Chapelle A (1997). Mutations predisposing to hereditary nonpolyposis colorectal cancer. *Advances in Cancer Research* **71**, 93–119

Powell SM, Zilz N, Beazer-Barclay Y *et al.* (1992). APC mutations occur early during colorectal tumorigenesis. *Nature* **359**, 235–237

Rabinovitch PS, Dziadon S, Brentnall TA *et al.* (1999). Pancolonic chromosomal instability precedes dysplasia and cancer in ulcerative colitis. *Cancer Research* **59**, 5148–5153

Rampino N, Yamamoto H, Ionov Y *et al.* (1997). Somatic frameshift mutations in the BAX gene in colon cancers of the microsatellite mutator phenotype. *Science* **275**, 967–969

Rashid A, Houlihan PS, Booker S *et al.* (2000). Phenotypic and molecular characteristics of hyperplastic polyposis. *Gastroenterology* **119**, 323–332

Riggins GJ, Thiagalingam S, Rozenblum E *et al.* (1996). Mad-related genes in the human. *Nature Genetics* **13**, 347–349

Sakamoto C (1998). Roles of COX-1 and COX-2 in gastrointestinal pathophysiology. *Journal of Gastroenterology* **33**, 618–624

Sakanaka C, Weiss JB, Williams LT (1998). Bridging of β-catenin and glycogen synthase kinase-3β by axin and inhibition of β-catenin-mediated transcription. *Proceedings of the National Academy of Sciences of the USA* **95**, 3020–3023

Sano H, Kawahito Y, Wilder RL *et al.* (1995). Expression of cyclooxygenase-1 and -2 in human colorectal cancer. *Cancer Research* **55**, 3785–3789

Shibata D, Peinado MA, Ionov Y *et al.* (1994). Genomic instability in repeated sequences is an early somatic event in colorectal tumorigenesis that persists after transformation. *Nature Genetics* **6**, 273–281

Shibata D, Reale MA, Lavin P *et al.* (1996). The DCC protein and prognosis in colorectal cancer [see comments]. *New England Journal of Medicine* **335**, 1727–1732

Souza RF, Appel R, Yin J *et al.* (1996). Microsatellite instability in the insulin-like growth factor II receptor gene in gastrointestinal tumours [letter] [published erratum appears in *Nature Genetics* 1996 **14**, 488]. *Nature Genetics* **14**, 255–257

Sparks AB, Morin PJ, Vogelstein B *et al.* (1998). Mutational analysis of the APC/β-catenin/Tcf pathway in colorectal cancer. *Cancer Research* **58**, 1130–1134

Spirio L, Olschwang S, Groden J *et al.* (1993). Alleles of the APC gene: an attenuated form of familial polyposis. *Cell* **75**, 951–957

Takagi Y, Kohmura H, Fukumura M *et al.* (1996). Somatic alterations of the DPC4 gene in human colorectal cancers in vivo [see comments]. *Gastroenterology* **111**, 1369–1372

Takaku K, Oshima M, Miyoshi H *et al.* (1998). Intestinal tumorigenesis in compound mutant mice of both Dpc4 (Smad4) and Apc genes. *Cell* **92**, 645–656

Tarmin L, Yin J, Harpaz N *et al.* (1995). Adenomatous polyposis coli gene mutations in ulcerative colitis-associated dysplasias and cancers versus sporadic colon neoplasms. *Cancer Research* **55**, 2035–2038

Tetsu O & McCormick F (1999). β-catenin regulates expression of cyclin D1 in colon carcinoma cells. *Nature* **398**, 422–426

Thiagalingam S, Lengauer C, Leach FS *et al.* (1996). Evaluation of candidate tumour suppressor genes on chromosome 18 in colorectal cancers. *Nature Genetics* **13**, 343–346

Thun MJ, Namboodiri MM, Heath CW Jr (1991). Aspirin use and reduced risk of fatal colon cancer [see comments]. *New England Journal of Medicine* **325**, 1593–1596

Tomlinson I & Bodmer W (1999). Selection, the mutation rate and cancer: ensuring that the tail does not wag the dog. *Nature Medicine* **5**, 11–12

Torlakovic E & Snover DC (1996). Serrated adenomatous polyposis in humans [see comments]. *Gastroenterology* **110**, 748–755

Triantafyllou K, Paspatis GA, Zizi A *et al*. (1999). p53 protein accumulation and colonic adenoma recurrence. *European Journal of Gastroenterology and Hepatology* **11**, 547–552

van der Luijt RB & van der Luijt PMK (1996). Protein truncation test for presymptomatic diagnosis of familial adenomatous polyposis. In Adolph K (ed.) *Methods in Molecular Genetics*. New York: Academic Press: pp 97–112

Vasen HF, van der Luijt RB, Slors JF *et al*. (1996a). Molecular genetic tests as a guide to surgical management of familial adenomatous polyposis [see comments]. *The Lancet* **348**, 433–435

Vasen HF, Wijnen JT, Menko FH *et al*. (1996b). Cancer risk in families with hereditary non-polyposis colorectal cancer diagnosed by mutation analysis [published erratum appears in *Gastroenterology* 1996 **111**, 1402]. *Gastroenterology* **110**, 1020–1027

Veale A (1965). *Intestinal Polyposis*. Cambridge: Cambridge University Press

Veigl ML, Kasturi L, Olechnowicz J *et al*. (1998). Biallelic inactivation of hMLH1 by epigenetic gene silencing, a novel mechanism causing human MSI cancers. *Proceedings of the National Academy of Sciences of the USA* **95**, 8698–8702

Vogelstein B, Fearon ER *et al*. (1988). Genetic alterations during colorectal-tumor development. *New England Journal of Medicine* **319**, 525–532

Walsh SV, Loda M, Torres CM *et al*. (1999). p53 and β catenin expression in chronic ulcerative colitis-associated polypoid dysplasia and sporadic adenomas: an immunohistochemical study. *American Journal of Surgical Pathology* **23**, 963–969

Wheeler JM, Beck NE, Kim HC *et al*. (1999). Mechanisms of inactivation of mismatch repair genes in human colorectal cancer cell lines: the predominant role of hMLH1. *Proceedings of the National Academy of Sciences of the USA* **96**, 10296–10301

Wijnen J, de Leeuw W, Vasen H *et al*. (1999). Familial endometrial cancer in female carriers of MSH6 germline mutations [letter]. *Nature Genetics* **23**, 142–144

Willenbucher RF, Zolman SF, Ferrell LD *et al*. (1997). Chromosomal alterations in ulcerative colitis-related neoplastic progression. *Gastroenterology* **113**, 791–801

Willenbucher RF, Aust DE, Chang CG *et al*. (1999). Genomic instability is an early event during the progression pathway of ulcerative-colitis-related neoplasia [see comments]. *American Journal of Pathology* **154**, 1825–1830

Williams CS, Luongo C, Bussey HS *et al*. (1996). Elevated cyclooxygenase-2 levels in Min mouse adenomas. *Gastroenterology* **111**, 1134–1140

Williams GT, Arthur JF, Radhika A *et al*. (1980). Metaplastic polyps and polyposis of the colorectum. *Histopathology* **4**, 155–170

Woodford-Richens K, Williamson J, Bevan S *et al*. (2000). Allelic loss at SMAD4 in polyps from juvenile polyposis patients and use of fluorescence in situ hybridization to demonstrate clonal origin of the epithelium. *Cancer Research* **60**, 2477–82

Woolf C (1958). A genetic study of carcinoma of the large intestine. *American Journal of Human Genetics* **10**, 42–47

Chapter 3

Cancer genetics and colorectal cancer: understanding how current data should be influencing routine clinical practice

Trevor Cole, Christopher Weiner and H Vicky Sleightholme

Introduction

Routine clinical practice provides the building blocks for any clinical service. Treatments and interventions aim to cure, alleviate symptoms or prevent disease from occurring in the first place. Clinicians supply a service by balancing the demands and wishes of their patients with what is effective and available. Healthcare commissioners face the task of balancing the funding of health care with healthcare need and demand across a whole range of services. Stevens and Raftery (1997) describe a model of the interrelationship of need, demand and supply in service provision (Figure 3.1 and Table 3.1). Using the definitions of 'need, demand and supply', seven separate service combinations can be identified (T Marshall, personal communication, 2000). These service situations are listed in Table 3.2.

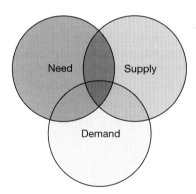

Figure 3.1 Venn diagram of demand, need and supply model of health care.

Combination 7 in Table 3.2 is the optimum area for any service provision. A central role of healthcare commissioners and clinicians is to increase the overlap of need, demand and supply. In this chapter we explore the current data on clinical genetics of colorectal cancer using the model of need, supply and demand to identify important

Table 3.1 Definition of need, demand and supply

Definitions	
Need	The ability to benefit from health care. This distinguishes it from 'neediness' which is a need for better health. The two essential elements of population need are, first, the incidence/ prevalence of a health problem and, second, the effectiveness/cost effectiveness of interventions available to deal with the problem
Demand	What people would be willing to pay for or might wish to use in a system of free health care
Supply	What is actually provided

Table 3.2 Possible patterns of need, demand and supply

1. Need, but no demand or supply
2. Demand, but no need or supply
3. Supply, but no need or demand
4. Need and demand, but no supply
5. Demand and supply, but no need
6. Need and supply, but no demand
7. Need, demand and supply

issues. We highlight not only what is known, but also areas of uncertainty and potential pitfalls. Thus, it will be possible to identify how current clinical practice may increase the overlap between the three areas and optimise service provision to the benefit of patients in a manner acceptable to both clinicians and healthcare commissioners.

Inherited mechanisms are believed to underlie between 5% and 30% of all colorectal cancers, most researchers believing that the figure lies somewhere towards the midpoint. Approximately 3–4% of cases of colorectal cancer are the result of distinct clinical syndromes (Table 3.3) (Burt 2000), familial adenomatous polyposis (FAP) and hereditary non-polyposis colon cancer (HNPCC) being the most common, for which the gene mutations have been identified. The remainder is recognised as familial clusters of colorectal cancer, which might be caused by undiscovered single gene inheritance, polygenic factors, multifactorial mechanisms, common environmental exposures or chance. The first group of distinct cancer syndromes is much less heterogeneous and more easily identified. Within this group is the strongest evidence that supply should be matched to needs. In particular, there is universal agreement that part of the management of FAP includes the proactive identification of 'at-risk' individuals so that surveillance and therapeutic intervention can facilitate a reduction in morbidity and mortality. The weight of evidence for such an interventionist approach in HNPCC and other single gene syndromes that predispose to colorectal cancer is less, but steadily accumulating, and most gastroenterologists, surgeons and clinical geneticists advocate a similar proactive approach.

Table 3.3 Table of single-gene colorectal cancer-predisposing syndromes, causative genes and surveillance strategy references

Syndrome	Causative gene(s)	CRC surveillance routinely recommended	References re phenotype and surveillance recommendations
Familial adenomatous polyposis (FAP)	APC	++	Vasen et al. (1990, 1997), Morton et al. (1993), Burt (2000)
Hereditary non-polyposis colorectal cancer (HNPCC)	MLH1, MSH2, MSH6, PMS1, PMS2, TGFβ	+	Vasen et al. (1993), Burt (2000), Chung (2000)
Juvenile polyposis	Smad4, DPC4, (PTEN)	+	Phillips et al. (1994), Scott-Conner et al. (1995), Burt (2000), Soravia et al. (2000)
Peutz–Jegher syndrome	STK11	+	Phillips et al. (1994), Burt (2000), Soravia et al. (2000)
Turcot's syndrome	APC, MMR	+	Phillips et al. (1994), Foulkes (1995), Burt (2000)
Cowden's syndrome/ PTEN mutation syndromes	PTEN	–	Phillips et al. (1994), Burt (2000)

TGFβ, transforming growth factor β.

The greatest variance of recommendations comes when considering familial clusters of colorectal cancer. Many patients and their doctors identify a 'demand' that has much weaker supporting evidence and shifts the balance further away from the 'ideals' of combination 7. If service provision has first to balance demands and supply, a potential conflict will arise with different thresholds of benefits being applied.

Our experience in the West Midlands, a mixed socioeconomic but geographically defined population of almost 5.3 million in central England, is that demand for colorectal cancer surveillance on the basis of family history is increasing. In many districts entry into surveillance is on an 'ad hoc' basis, similar to that identified by Scholfield et al. (1998), which has resulted in some districts having an abundance of 'lower' increased risk cases outnumbering, and potentially having a detrimental affect on, the supply of service for symptomatic patients and individuals at greater risk. On the basis of our own experience in the West Midlands, we have proposed a more universal approach to 'inclusion guidelines' for colorectal cancer surveillance using reported family history. This has slowed the exponential increase in numbers of screened patients but has identified a higher risk cohort. This has the potential to provide a more equitable service provision based on need and the ability collect more meaningful data on the cost consequences and benefit, and therefore in the longer term facilitate the matching of need, demand and supply.

Clinical patterns of familial colon cancer and surveillance strategies

Familial adenomatous polyposis

Familial adenomatous polyposis is an autosomal dominant genetic condition predisposing, in almost 100% of gene carriers, to the development of hundreds or thousands of adenomatous colonic polyps and colorectal cancer (Bulow 1987). Colonic polyps are identifiable in 50% of gene carriers by age 14 and the mean age of colorectal cancer is about 40 years (Burn *et al.* 1991; Foulkes 1995). It accounts for approximately 1% of colorectal cancer and has an incidence of 1 in 8,000 (Foulkes 1995). The causative gene, adenomatous polyposis coli (*APC*), was cloned in 1991 (Kinzler *et al.* 1991; Nishisho *et al.* 1991) and enables molecular identification of gene carriers in approximately 70–80% of families (Foulkes 1995). Further studies of the *APC* gene has shown that some mutations in the 5′-region can sometimes result in an attenuated phenotype (AFAP) with fewer than a 100 polyps, later age of tumour development and non-penetrance in some gene carriers (Foulkes 1995). Mutations throughout most of the gene can result in extracolonic manifestations and, although there are some genotype–phenotype correlations, these are not always predictable (Foulkes 1995). Many of these instances would previously have been called Gardener's syndrome and some of the additional tumour complications of FAP are summarised in Table 3.4.

Table 3.4 Early and late extracolonic tumours in familial adenomatous polyposis (FAP)

Hepatoblastoma (early)
Mandibular osteomas (early or late)
Adrenal adenoma (early or late)
Desmoid disease (early or late)
Brain tumours (early or late)
Papillary thyroid cancer (late – mostly females)
Periampullary carcinoma (late)

After the diagnosis of FAP, a full family history should be taken, although approximately 30% of cases represent 'new' mutations and no other affected member will be identified. It is recommended that siblings and offspring should be offered annual flexible sigmoidoscopy between the ages of 12 and 40, or until proven not to be a gene carrier with molecular predictive testing. Examination of parents of apparently 'new' cases should include at least a single examination. It has been suggested that this should be a colonoscopy to prevent missing AFAP.

In families with identified mutations, molecular testing should be carried out before surveillance begins at around 12–14 years. There is controversy about whether such testing should always be delayed to immediately before instigation of surveillance or whether there could be justification to bring this forward to early childhood at parental request. Current studies looking at the psychological implications and impact of testing at different ages in childhood are in progress (Michie *et al.* 2000).

Evidence from several sources has shown that proactive intervention, molecular investigation and surveillance can reduce both morbidity and mortality in gene carriers with FAP (Vasen *et al.* 1990; Burn *et al.* 1991; Morton *et al.* 1993; Bapat *et al.* 1999) (Table 3.5). Once polyps have been identified, the timing and type of surgery available should be discussed with the patient. This is likely to be a particularly sensitive subject with teenagers and young adults. The two most common surgical options are ileal–rectal anastomosis, with subsequent rectal surveillance or reconstruction of a rectal pouch using the terminal small bowel. If an ileal–rectal anastomosis is performed, it may well be that an ileostomy or pouch will subsequently be required. There is now evidence that the surgical management choices may well be influenced by the nature of the mutation. Mutations in the second part of the gene (after codon 1250) are associated with a more severe phenotype and therefore a greater likelihood of earlier definitive surgery or a subsequent cancer. In this group, a restorative colectomy may be preferred as the initial surgery despite the greater frequency of surgery-related symptoms (Vasen *et al.* 1996a).

A European multicentre study (concerted action in polyposis prevention – CAPP) is currently examining the role of chemoprophylaxis using agents such as aspirin and/or non-digestible starch (Burn *et al.* 1995).

Post-colectomy there remains a residual risk of malignant disease, in particular papillary thyroid cancer and periampullary carcinoma. The latter has raised questions about the role of upper gastrointestinal endoscopy. Several authors and speciality subgroups have advocated regular upper gastrointestinal endoscopy and even preventive pancreatic surgery (King *et al.* 2000). However, the proportion of cases with duodenal polyposis that go on to carcinoma appears to be relatively small (< 5%) (Vasen *et al.* 1997; Sondegaard *et al.* 1999) and unpredictable. Furthermore, an aggressive surgical approach has resulted only in a mean increase in survival of 7 months in affected individuals (Vasen *et al.* 1997). Overall the role of upper gastrointestinal endoscopy needs further evaluation.

Hereditary non-polyposis colon cancer

In 1913 Warthin described a large kindred with both colorectal cancer and gynaecological tumours. The family was reviewed in two subsequent papers by Warthin and, together with a paper from Lynch and colleagues in 1966, formed the basis of a condition that became known as HNPCC or Lynch syndrome. Extensive epidemiological, clinical and molecular investigation has clarified many of the features and Lynch *et al.* (1993) provided an excellent review of the subject.

Table 3.5 West Midlands FAP register data on surveillance effectiveness

Method of identification	Total	Mean (range) age at diagnosis (years)	Dukes' classification					Multiple	Patients with colorectal cancer
			A	B	C	'D'	Unknown		
Screening	51	23.6 (10–48)	1	1	0	0	1	1	3
Symptoms	53	38.5 (12–58)	0	10	13	5	6	7	34
Unknown	3	–	–	–	–	–	–	–	0
Total	107		1	11	13	5	7	8	37

Data from Morton et al. (1993).

In 1991, a research collaboration defined clinical criteria to facilitate consistency in their work and these became known as the Amsterdam criteria. Applying strict Amsterdam criteria, Evans *et al.* (1997) reported that HNPCC accounted for less than 2% of colorectal cancers. Since 1991, the criteria have been modified by several groups (Tables 3.6 and 3.7) and further clinical and molecular studies suggest that, if the modified criteria are used, HNPCC represents between 3% and 5% of colorectal cancers (Syngal *et al.* 2000).

Table 3.6 Amsterdam criteria

Three or more cases of colorectal cancer
In a minimum of two generations
One affected individual first degree of the other two cases of colorectal cancer
One case diagnosed before the age of 50
FAP excluded

Table 3.7 Subsequent modification to Amsterdam criteria

Modified Amsterdam	Amsterdam II	Bethesda
To adjust for small families – can include just two cases of colorectal cancer (one < 55)	As Amsterdam criteria but can substitute other HNPCC-related tumours, e.g. endometrial, small bowel, renal tract transitional cell cancer	Amsterdam criteria
		Patient with any two HNPCC-related cancers
Two colorectal cancers and either endometrial cancer or other early onset cancer		Two first-degree relatives with HNPCC-related cancers, one < 45 years or adenoma, < 40 years
		Patient with colorectal cancer or endometrial cancer < 45 years
		Specific colorectal cancer histology, < 45 years
		Adenoma, < 40 years

Modified from review by Syngal *et al.* (2000).

The spectrum and frequency of tumours in HNPCC remain controversial. In a British study, which attempted to collect an unbiased sample by working back from an unselected cohort of early onset colorectal cancers, the spectrum of tumours illustrated in Figure 3.2 was identified (Dunlop *et al.* 1997). Other series have produced slightly different, often higher, incidences for these tumours but may be influenced by ascertainment bias.

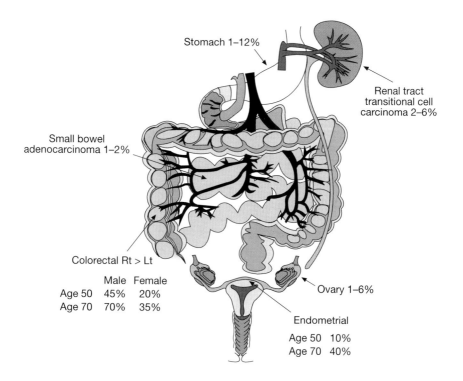

Stomach 1–12%

Renal tract transitional cell carcinoma 2–6%

Small bowel adenocarcinoma 1–2%

Colorectal Rt > Lt

	Male	Female
Age 50	45%	20%
Age 70	70%	35%

Ovary 1–6%

Endometrial

Age 50	10%
Age 70	40%

Figure 3.2 Tumour spectrum and incidence in hereditary non-polyposis colorectal cancer (HNPCC). Range of tumour incidence from selected papers (upper figures may be overestimates as a result of selection bias)

A series of molecular papers report the cloning of six different causative genes. Five of theses genes (*MSH2*, *MSH6*, *MLH1*, *PMS1* and *PMS2*) appear to be involved in DNA repair processes (Chung 2000). At a somatic level this will often be identified by the presence of additional bands on gel electrophoresis from errors or slippage in tumour (but not blood), or DNA amplification of mono- or dinucleotide repeat alleles (Figure 3.3) (Chung 2000). This process appears to occur only after function of both copies of the relevant repair gene has been lost in line with the Knudson two-hit hypothesis of tumour-suppressor genes (Knudson 1971).

Guidelines for surveillance in HNPCC have been suggested by several groups and differ significantly in the spectrum of tumours sites monitored, the frequency recommended and methodology used (Hodgson *et al.* 1995; Vasen *et al.* 1996b; Weber 1996; Burke *et al.* 1997; Burt 2000). Surveillance strategies for extracolonic sites show the greatest variation and not surprisingly the least evidence of benefit has been gathered for them.

It is now almost universally accepted that colonoscopy rather than barium enema should be the method of surveillance. However, failure to reach the caecum at

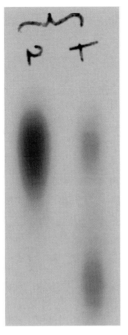

Figure 3.3 Molecular analysis of blood (germline DNA – lane N) versus tumour DNA (somatic DNA – lane T) from a patient with early onset colorectal cancer showing microsatellite instability (MSI) in tumour tissue.

colonoscopy may be an indication for barium enema because there is a greater proportion of right-sided tumours in HNPCC (Vasen *et al.* 1993; Chung 2000). The age at which screening should begin has gradually been decreasing as anecdotal reports of earlier cases occur. Previous guidelines, which suggested beginning surveillance at age 30–35, have been replaced with recommendations for initiating colonoscopies at 25 or even 20 years in some reviews (Vasen *et al.* 1996b; Weber 1996; Burke *et al.* 1997; Burt 2000). Data showing benefit for surveillance at these younger ages have yet to be collected, and even starting at age 20 will not alter the morbidity or mortality of one or two unpredictable extreme variations within families.

A similar balance exists between the optimal frequency of bowel examinations. Previous suggestions of 3-yearly colonoscopies have been modified to 2-yearly or less, often on the basis of anecdotal reports of interval tumours (Vasen *et al.* 1993). This report needs to be judged against the early tumour stage of all six interval tumours (Dukes' A or B) and the likelihood that some of these carcinomas would not have had detectable tubulovillous adenomas, and possibly presented as would have adenocarcinomas irrespective of screening interval. The greater frequency of surveillance may also have potential disadvantages, extending beyond the cost and its impact on other colorectal services. They include a greater risk of complications and the potential to increase the rate of non-compliance within some patient groups. Until clear evidence of benefit of one surveillance interval can be provided, it is likely that the broad range of 12- to 36-monthly intervals will be applied. This will probably be modified by circumstances such as the patient's age, degree of risk (e.g. whether at 50% or 25% risk), patient compliance and the availability of resources (Vasen *et al.* 1996b; Weber 1996; Burke *et al.* 1997; Burt 2000). For a number of asymptomatic gene carriers, or individuals with only small polyps, prophylactic colectomy is becoming an option that they may consider (Vasen *et al.* 1996b; Burke *et al.* 1997).

For females in HNPCC families, with proven mismatch repair gene mutations, the lifetime risk of endometrial adenocarcinoma is at least 40% and probably exceeds the risk of colorectal cancer (Dunlop *et al.* 1997). Management strategies have included annual transvaginal ultrasonography and/or annual endometrial biopsy. Transvaginal ultrasonography, in premenopausal women, is of debatable benefit and probably justified only because it may allow additional ovarian assessment (Ayhan *et al.* 1992; Lynch *et al.* 1992; Burke *et al.* 1997). Ovarian cancer is also more frequent in HNPCC, either as a distinct entity or as a synchronous endometrial cancer. The presence of endometrial hyperplasia is not a good predictor of subsequent malignant change and the 5-year survival rate for endometrial adenocarcinoma is better than 80% in women aged below 65 (West Midlands Health Authority 1995), which would be true of most endometrial tumours diagnosed in HNPCC. Therefore, improving survival by surveillance will be difficult. It is also important to note that there is no published study of outcome for endometrial surveillance in women at increased risk, based on a history of confirmed HNPCC. One alternative approach frequently pursued by female gene carriers is hysterectomy with bilateral oophorectomy, which will obviously have the greatest effect on risk reduction, but again lacks supporting data on overall survival (Vasen *et al.* 1996b; Burke *et al.* 1997).

The role of gynaecological surveillance and/or surgery in families fulfilling clinical criteria for HNPCC, but with no identified mutations, raises even greater uncertainties. The risk of gynaecological cancers is unknown in these families but is probably lower than in families known to have mutations, especially in the absence of a family history of such tumours. Once again a wide variety of guidelines have been proposed, but none with data to show a proven benefit (Vasen *et al.* 1996b; Burke *et al.* 1997; Burt 2000). One pragmatic approach is suggested in the West Midlands Family Cancer Strategy outlined below (Cole & Sleightholme 2000). Invariably there is likely to be some variation in the approach, based on individual discussions within families and influenced by patient anxiety and compliance.

Currently, two papers have attempted to address the potential benefit from colonoscopic surveillance in HNPCC (Jarvinen *et al.* 1995; Vasen *et al.* 1998). Unfortunately, neither study is randomised, and a new study with a 'no treatment' arm would probably be resisted by patients and possibly ethical committees. However, the papers of Jarvinen *et al.* (1995) and Vasen *et al.* (1998) combined provide circumstantial evidence supporting a role for surveillance in reducing morbidity, mortality and cost to the health service.

In 1995, Jarvinen *et al.* showed a significantly lower incidence of cancer, over a 10-year period, in a cohort of individuals at a 50% risk of carrying an *HNPCC* gene who opted for 3-yearly colonoscopic surveillance, compared with a cohort who declined this input. There was also a non-significant reduction in cancer-related deaths in the screened group. Logically, one would assume that the benefit would be greater as surveillance continued longer and more patients passed through ages associated with a greater risk of cancer. Furthermore, since the study, a number of *HNPCC* genes have been identified and a proportion of individuals (probably > 50%) in such families will be excluded by virtue of not being a gene carrier in both the screened and unscreened group. This would probably increase the significance assuming that most cancers occurred in gene carriers rather than as phenocopies.

In 1998, using data from the Dutch HNPCC register, Vasen *et al.* looked at cost-effectiveness modelling analyses for screening and tumour prevention in gene carriers against the cost of management in unscreened symptomatic gene carriers. Using different models of penetrance and prevention, all analyses appear to show evidence of increased life expectancy and a reduction of cost in favour of surveillance for at-risk patients. This, together with the data from Jarvinen and patient demand, seems to provide consistent evidence in favour of colonic surveillance. However, the precise protocol to be implemented has yet to be defined and is currently based on 'local expert interpretation' of the published protocols (Hodgson *et al.* 1995; Vasen *et al.* 1996b; Weber 1996; Burke *et al.* 1997; Burt 2000).

Other autosomal dominant colon cancer disorders

There are several autosomal dominant colorectal predisposing syndromes and these are listed in Table 3.3. In all the listed examples the penetrance of colorectal cancer appears to be lower than in FAP or HNPCC, but are also associated with an increased tumour risk at other sites. Specific groups have suggested guidelines for surveillance in these conditions, but this is based on fewer data than in FAP or HNPCC, in terms of the colorectal cancer risk and benefit. Evidence for surveillance recommendation is also lacking for other sites, but the reader is referred to the reviews referenced in Table 3.3 (Phillips *et al.* 1994; Scott-Conner *et al.* 1995; Foulkes 1995; Burt 2000; Soravia *et al.* 2000).

Familial clustering of colorectal cancer of unknown aetiology

Familial clusters of colorectal cancer exist that do not meet the Amsterdam criteria or have an identified DNA mismatch repair (*MMR*) gene mutation, and as a result are not classified as HNPCC. It has been evident for many years that such a family history of colorectal cancer is associated with significantly increased risk of a similar tumour in first-degree relatives (Woolf 1958; Lovett 1976; Søndergaard *et al.* 1991; St John *et al.* 1993). These series also showed that, the younger the age of onset of the colorectal cancer or the more extensive the family history, the greater the increase in the relative risk. Such data can be used to provide risk stratification in patient cohorts and management guidelines (Houlston *et al.* 1990). However, the underlying aetiology of the elevated risk will remain unknown in individual patients or families. Plausible explanations include coincidental clustering, shared predisposing environmental exposures, multifactorial interactions between environmental and genetic factors, and genes with lower penetrance than seen with *APC* or the *MMR* genes.

Larger families will also appear to be at an increased risk by virtue of the coincidental occurrence of tumours in larger 'at-risk' family cohorts. This is the result of fixed denominator data based around generations, and variable nominator data made up of the individual family members. Demographic changes mean that we live in an ageing population and, as colorectal cancer remains primarily a disease of elderly people, the overall incidence of colorectal cancer is increasing. This could result in greater numbers of families having a documented family history than in previous generations. This may be particularly problematic with the late-onset cases which are least likely to have a genetic component, but are likely to be increasingly recognised and potentially have the least benefit from early surveillance. Unpublished data from an unselected cohort of colorectal cancer follow-up patients in the West Midlands confirmed that over a quarter had a first-degree relative with colorectal cancer, but that this appeared to be biased towards large families.

Data have been drawn from a number of sources, including the potential benefits of surveillance in FAP and HNPCC, and epidemiological papers identifying the risk in relatives of colon cancer cases, and subsequently extrapolated to develop screening strategies for colorectal cancer in many families with much less significant family histories. These individuals also represent the average of this group and all or much of any benefit might be the result of a small proportion of cases at higher risk.

Guidelines from the USA frequently advocate population surveillance of individuals over the age of 50 (Burt 2000; Rex *et al.* 2000). In addition, surveillance for people with a family history of bowel cancer is advocated both earlier and in many cases more intensively than in the average risk population (Burt 2000; Rex *et al.* 2000). Despite intensive and protracted clinical and literature reviews, it has been difficult to provide a unified surveillance proposal for this 'at-risk' group.

The American College of Gastroenterologists made specific recommendations, but point out that one of the participating group, the Agency for Healthcare Policy and Research (AHCPR), was unable to identify which of the suggested options were optimal (Rex *et al.* 2000).

Possible model for familial cancer management

Colorectal cancer is not alone in showing a significant increased referral rate for management advice after the identification of a family history of cancer. Indeed, the number of patients with a family history of breast cancer exceeds colorectal referrals by a factor of 3 or 4 in many genetic departments or cancer units in the UK. This is despite the fact that epidemiological data would suggest that approximately equal numbers of patients would be expected to have a genetic susceptibility to these two tumour sites. There is also significantly more circumstantial evidence for a potential benefit from colorectal surveillance compared with breast surveillance in these settings.

Primary care practitioners are frequently asked advice concerning a family history of cancer and have difficulty identifying the most pertinent points or providing consistent advice across or between families. The West Midlands experience is of an increasing demand at all levels of the healthcare system. The changing referral pattern of common solid tumours to the West Midlands Genetics service for the last decade is presented in Figure 3.4. Pilot data from one health district showed that this under-represented by a factor of four- or fivefold the number of cases referred on to colorectal or breast care teams and with an even greater, but unknown, workload impact on primary care (see Figures 3.3 and 3.4). To address these referral pressures we devised a triage approach and named the West Midlands Family Cancer Strategy (WMFACS) (www.bham.ac.uk/ich/clingen.htm) (Cole & Sleightholme 2000).

West Midlands Family Cancer Strategy

An algorithm for the strategy is provided at the website given above.

A patient seeking advice about their family history of cancer is requested by the GP to complete a data collection form (www.bham.ac.uk/ich/clingen.htm). This can be given to the patient to take away so that they can confer with other family members. This has meant that family information, and hence histology, was more likely to be obtained, resulting in more accurate advice being given to the patient in the clinic. Studies by House *et al.* (1999) and Aitken *et al.* (1995) showed respectively that a questionnaire approach was acceptable to patients and usually accurate.

The inclusion criteria for referral and explanation are provided on the same form, so these are always available to the GP and patient with the form. Most GPs had requested that this information was easily available to the patients because they felt that in most cases it provided additional reassurance. The form also acts as a referral letter, saving time and providing very full details.

To provide consistency of management and to facilitate data collection, cases requiring referral are forwarded directly to the cancer co-ordinator based in the Clinical Genetics Unit (CGU) or through identified clinicians in cancer units. The co-ordinator alone requests confirmation of all histology, once consent is obtained, thus preventing duplication within families. Three years of pilot data have been collected

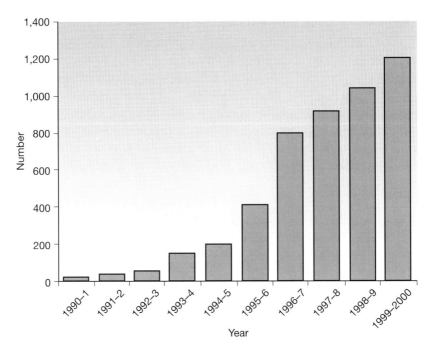

Figure 3.4 Cancer referrals to the West Midlands Regional Genetics Cancer Service in the last 10 years.

from Herefordshire, catchment population of 175,000, after the model has been rigidly applied at a primary care level. A subsidiary study in inner city Birmingham showed that almost 80% of patients replied after one or two reminders were sent. Follow-up of a subset of the non-responders showed that the majority either recognised that they did not meet the referral criteria on the form, and therefore did not complete their details, or did not wish to proceed with the referral. In all cases the referring doctor for non-responders was informed that the patient had not been seen.

Once available information had been collected, all forms were reviewed and processed by consultants within the CGU according to protocol guidelines (see website mentioned above). A standard letter was sent to the GP summarising the outcome of the form review.

A 3-year pilot study identified that overall referral, because of a family history of cancer, fell by over 50% (Figure 3.5) and patients requiring surveillance by even more (Figure 3.6). However, the proportion of patients in high-risk categories rose, particularly noticeably in patients with a significant risk of colorectal cancer. The overall effect was that the ratio of colorectal cancer to breast cancer referrals came closer to parity as would be expected on epidemiological grounds. The relative ratio of colon to breast cancer case referrals rose from approximately 1 : 5 to 1 : 1.6.

As the potential greater benefit is likely to come from colorectal cancer surveillance, this was a positive change in referral pattern.

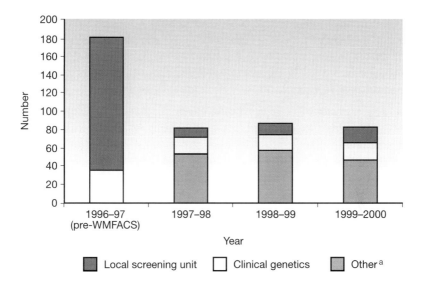

Figure 3.5 Absolute referral rate of cancer genetic cases following implementation of the WMFACS in Herefordshire, and comparison pre-implementation with referrals to cancer unit and clinical genetics. [a]Represents forms received but not referred on to screening units or clinical genetics.

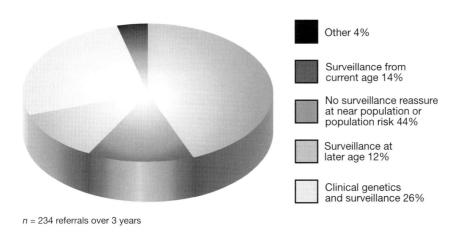

n = 234 referrals over 3 years

Figure 3.6 Proportion of referrals into WMFACS in Herefordshire requiring active surveillance.

Discussion

Clinicians and healthcare commissioners face the difficult task of balancing the supply of health care with the needs and demands of individuals and populations. In an ideal world, there would be no resource constraints to meet people's needs and demands. However, in the light of scarcity it is unethical to fail to consider the opportunity cost and efficiency of various packages of health care. Therefore, as the information on proven benefits is limited, we have to look towards pragmatic approaches to balance needs, demands and supply.

The complex phenomenon of healthcare demand is generated through the interaction of wants, knowledge, expectations, fears, advertising, the broader socioeconomic environment and of course 'need'. A common mistake is to equate demand for a service with the need for a service, without considering all the other influences upon the aforementioned demand. This may be acceptable in a purely consumerist-driven healthcare system, but is unlikely to be appropriate in the UK, or similar countries, which provide health care free at the point of access, paid out of taxes. However, there is substantial demand for cancer genetics health care in the West Midlands, and this is likely to continue rising as our knowledge of the underlying genetics of disease improves. This raises the question of how one manages this demand to ensure that need is met efficiently. In colorectal cancer the need is likely to be fixed in the short term while demand continues to rise. Therefore, to meet the need for cancer genetic services in an efficient manner, it is essential to look at the supply of clinical services.

There is a gradient of risk for the development of colorectal cancer in an individual, depending on underlying genetic and environmental influences. The natural result of such a gradient is that one individual may potentially benefit from a particular healthcare package, whereas another individual, with a different risk profile, based on the interaction of genetic and environmental factors, may not benefit from the same care. For colorectal cancer, we have the ability to separate some clinically distinct groups of genetic or genetic/environmental diseases such as FAP, HNPCC, other dominantly inherited conditions, familial clusters and coincidental tumours. In future, as a result of advances through the human genome project, further subgroups will be identified resolving the grey areas that lie between these clinical classifications. The collection of further data on healthcare interventions will allow more precise targeting at people who can potentially benefit. However, in the meantime it would be wrong to ignore our present knowledge and understanding to develop healthcare services for colorectal cancer.

There are a number of potential service provision models that could be supplied to manage the demand for colorectal cancer genetic services:

- An absolute ban on the provision of any services relating to colorectal cancer genetics. This would ignore present knowledge and is almost certainly unacceptable to most individuals.

- Implementation of a population screening programme that would actively invite people into the service. This may be adopted in the future, but current resources and knowledge make this inappropriate, especially while any harm, at individual and population level, remains unquantified.
- Individual medical practitioners could be asked to decide on patient management requests, as is the most common current practice. The colorectal cancer risk of people demanding services would range from close to 100%, e.g. known FAP gene carriers, to individuals at approximately population risk. Variation between medical practitioners, and even within a single individual, could exaggerate service inequalities and modify unwittingly the ability to benefit. Furthermore, if such service provision results in inefficient use of resources this could be to the detriment of the remaining population.
- A triage service to filter those least likely to benefit from screening ensures that available healthcare resources, such as colonoscopy screening, are targeted at those with the greatest potential need and none is treated inequitably compared with their 'risk cohort'. This system promotes efficiency in resource utilisation, maximises any potential benefits and minimises potential harms for those requesting active management for elevated colorectal cancer risk.

In FAP, few people would argue against the need to ensure surveillance and treatment options for at-risk individuals. Failure to provide adequate healthcare packages will result in most gene carriers presenting with late-stage disease. The management options for FAP in affected or at-risk individuals have low morbidity and mortality risks, and intervention options are broadly acceptable to the relevant patient group. Although a few areas are still open to debate, such as the timing of molecular testing and the management of extracolonic manifestations, FAP displays the most extensive overlap of need, demand and supply as described in the model by Stevens and Raftery (1997).

HNPCC forms the next most clearly defined group of genetic colorectal cancer. The evidence strongly suggests a potential need that can be met by increased surveillance. Jarvinen *et al.* (1995) showed a statistically significant difference in the incidence of colon cancer in people receiving screening. The lower cancer-related mortality did not reach statistical significance. Despite weaknesses such as self-selection to surveillance in the study, there is a substantial belief of benefit which may make it difficult to argue for future randomised control trials. The degree of resistance to such studies is likely to differ greatly between public health physicians and clinicians managing individual patients.

Vasen *et al.* (1998) carried out economic modelling of cost-effectiveness for surveillance in hypothetical gene carriers in known HNPCC families, and suggested that screening affected individuals was beneficial and cost-effective. However, the modelling assumed that every patient would follow suggested care pathways and did not include the mechanism or cost underlying case identification. Therefore, it cannot yet be used to justify a proactive case identification programme in the general population although it does strengthen the case that surveillance for families with HNPCC is beneficial. Questions remain over precise screening protocols for colorectal cancer, and the management of extracolonic manifestations is unproven. In view of these uncertainties in the management of HNPCC, it is still important to ensure that reliable data on effectiveness are collected for all tumour sites. If randomised trials on many of these aspects are considered unethical, collaboration between national and international groups to facilitate careful observation and audit of clinical practice is vital.

The familial clusters of colorectal cancer are the least clearly defined group that may benefit from increased surveillance over and above that offered to the general population. Burt (2000), in an excellent and substantive review of the US perspective, notes that cost, inconvenience and risk may be factors against a population colonoscopy programme. However, in view of the same lack of evidence concerning the optimal surveillance programme in moderately increased risk cohorts, his statement that randomised studies may be unethical seems unfounded at the current time.

Such extensive surveillance programmes can have significant cost and health service implications to the provision in other areas of colorectal or general gastroenterological service. With potentially less significant increases in lifetime colorectal cancer risk, the ratio of complications to benefit increases. Furthermore, such programmes may induce increased levels of patient anxiety and false negatives lead to inappropriate reassurance. Therefore, although this is a group for whom surveillance may be indicated, the nature and cost of this need careful evaluation, a point stressed by Dunlop and Campbell (1997).

The results of several large population studies of average-risk patients may provide an appropriate benchmark for subsequent randomised studies in patients with a moderately increased risk of colorectal cancer. Perhaps we should argue that failure to attempt to collect data on cost consequence and effectiveness for patients undergoing surveillance is at least as pressing an ethical argument as that made by Burt (2000).

A system that filters out people with the least potential to benefit from interventions, and aimed at patients with an increased risk of colorectal cancer, has been developed in the West Midlands region. It draws upon the present limited knowledge relating to the genetics of colon cancer. The current data from the pilot study do indeed suggest that such a system has the desired effect on demand management for familial cancer services. Referral and overall surveillance decreased, and resources were concentrated on those at highest risk and therefore potentially those with the greatest chance of benefit from such a service. However, it has not been proved whether or not such a system actually delivers improvements in morbidity and mortality for those entering the service. Many aspects are still open to debate, such as those relating to the intervention options in HNPCC, and more wide-ranging uncertainties in familial clustering of colorectal cancer. However, demand is being managed rationally according to potential ability to benefit and systems are in place to facilitate monitoring results. We suggest that this pragmatic approach uses current data to influence clinical practice to the benefit of clinicians, health service managers and the population. Although we support the implementation of management strategies in line with many of the recommendations referenced in the text for FAP and HNPCC, this should include data collection and evaluation. This is of even greater importance for familial clusters of colorectal cancer, and we would suggest that surveillance should not be undertaken unless clinicians are willing to collect the data to allow ongoing reassessment.

References

Aitken J, Bain C, Ward M *et al.* (1995). How accurate is self-reported family history of colorectal cancer? *American Journal of Epidemiology* **141**, 863–871

Ayhan A, Yalcin OT, Selcuk Tuncer Z *et al.* (1992) Synchronous primary malignancies of the female genital tract. *European Journal of Obstetrics and Gynaecology and Reproductive Biology* **45**, 63–66

Bapat B, Noorani H, Cohen Z *et al.* (1999). Cost comparison of predictive testing versus conventional clinical surveillance for familial adenomatous polyposis. *Gut* **44**, 698–703

Bulow S (1987). Familial adenomatous polyposis. *Danish Medical Journal* **34**, 1–15

Burke W, Petersen G, Lynch P *et al.* (1997). Recommendations for follow-up care of individuals with an inherited predisposition to cancer: 1 Hereditary nonpolyposis colon cancer. *Journal of the American Medical Association* **277**, 915–919

Burn J, Chapman P, Delhanty J *et al.* (1991). The UK northern region genetic register for familial adenomatous polyposis coli: use of age of onset, CHRPE, and DNA markers in risk calculations. *Journal of Medical Genetics* **28**, 289–296

Burn J, Chapman PD, Mathers J *et al.* (1995). The protocol for a European double blind trial of aspirin and resistant starch in familial adenomatous polyposis: the CAPP study. *European Journal of Cancer* **31A**, 1385–1386

Burt RW (2000). Colon cancer screening. *Gastroenterology* **119**, 837–853

Chung DC (2000). The genetic basis of colorectal cancer: insights into critical pathways of tumorigenesis. *Gastroenterology* **119**, 854–865

Cole TRP & Sleightholme HV (2000) ABC of colorectal cancer: the role of clinical genetics in management. *British Medical Journal* **321**, 943–946

Dunlop M & Campbell H (1997). Screening for people with a family history of colorectal cancer. *British Medical Journal* **314**, 1779–1780

Dunlop MG, Farrington SM, Carothers AD *et al.* (1997). Cancer risk associated with germline DNA mismatch repair gene mutations. *Human Molecular Genetics* **6**, 105–110

Evans DG, Walsh S, Jeacock J *et al.* (1997). Incidence of hereditary non-polyposis colorectal cancer in a population-based study of 1137 consecutive cases of colorectal cancer. *British Journal of Surgery* **84**, 1281–1285

Foulkes WD (1995). A tale of four syndromes: familial adenomatous polyposis, Gardner syndrome, attenuated APC and Turcot syndrome. *Quarterly Journal of Medicine* **88**, 853–863

Hodgson SV, Bishop DT, Dunlop MG *et al*. (1995). Suggested screening guidelines for familial colorectal cancer. *Journal of Medical Screening* **2**, 45–51

Houlston RS, Murday V, Harcocopos C *et al*. (1990). Screening and genetic counselling for relatives of patients with colorectal cancer in a family cancer clinic. *British Medical Journal* **301**, 366–368

House W, Sharp D, Sheridan E (1999). Identifying and screening patients at high risk of colorectal cancer in general practice. *Journal of Medical Screening* **6**, 205–208

Jarvinen HJ, Mecklin JP, Sistonen P (1995) Screening reduces colorectal cancer rate in families with hereditary nonpolyposis colorectal cancer. *Gastroenterology* **108**, 1405–1411

King JE, Dozios RR, Lindor NM *et al*. (2000). Care of patients and their families with familial adenomatous polyposis. *Mayo Clinic Proceedings* **75**, 57–67

Kinzler KW, Nilbert MC, Su LK *et al*. (1991). Identification of FAP locus genes on chromosome 5q21. *Science* **253**, 661–665

Knudson AG (1971). Mutation and cancer: statistical study of retinoblastoma. *Proceedings of the National Academy of Sciences of the USA* **68**, 820–823

Lovett E. (1976). Family studies in cancer of the colon and rectum. *British Journal of Surgery* **63**, 13–18

Lynch HT, Shaw MW, Magnuson CW *et al*. (1966). Hereditary factors in two large midwestern kindreds. *Archives of Internal Medicine* **117**, 206–212

Lynch HT, Cavalieri RJ, Lynch JF *et al*. (1992) Gynecologic cancer clues to Lynch syndrome II: a family report. *Gynecological Oncology* **44**, 198–203

Lynch HT, Smyrk TC, Watson P *et al*. (1993). Genetics, natural history, tumour spectrum and pathology of hereditary nonpolyposis colorectal cancer: an updated review. *Gastroenterology* **104**, 1535–1549

Michie S, Marteau T, Armstrong D *et al*. (2000). Predictive genetic testing in children and adults: a study of emotional impact. *Journal of Medical Genetics* **37**(suppl 1), SP21A

Morton DG, Macdonald F, Haydon J, Cullen R, Barker G (1993). Screening practice for familial adenomatous polyposis: the potential for regional registers. *British Journal of Surgery* **80**, 255–258

Nishisho I, Nakamura Y, Miyoshi Y *et al*. (1991). Mutations of chromosome 5q21 genes in FAP and colorectal cancer patients. *Science* **253**, 665–9

Phillips RKS, Spigelman AD, Thomson JPS, eds (1994). *Familial Adenomatous Polyposis and other Polyposis Syndromes*. London: Edward Arnold

Rex DK, Johhnson DA, Lieberman DA *et al*. (2000). Colorectal cancer prevention 2000: screening recommendations of the American college of gastroenterology. *American Journal of Gastroenterology* **95**, 868–877

St John DJB, McDermott FT, Hopper JL *et al*. (1993). Cancer risk in relatives of patients with common colorectal cancer. *Annals of Internal Medicine* **118**, 785–790

Scholfield JH, Johnson AG, Shorthouse AJ (1998). Current surgical practice in screening for colorectal cancer based on family history criteria. *British Journal of Surgery* **85**, 1543–1546

Scott-Conner CEH, Hausmann M, Hall TJ *et al*. (1995). Familial juvenile polyposis: patterns of recurrence and implications for surgical management. *Journal of the American College of Surgeons* **181**, 407–413

Sondegaard Galle T, Juel K, Bulow S (1999). Causes of death in familial adenomatous polyposis. *Scandinavian Journal of Gastroenterology* **34**, 808–812

Søndergaard JO, Bulow S, Lynge E (1991). Cancer incidence among parents of patients with colorectal cancer. *International Journal of Cancer* **47**, 202–206

Soravia C, Berk T, Cohen Z (2000). Genetic testing and surgical decision making in hereditary colorectal cancer. International *Journal of Colorectal Disease* **15**, 21–28

Stevens A & Raftery J, eds (1997). *Health Care Needs and Assessment: The epidemiologically based needs assessment reviews.* Oxford: Radcliffe Medical Press

Syngal S, Fox EA, Eng C *et al.* (2000). Sensitivity and specificity of clinical criteria for hereditary non-polyposis colorectal cancer associated mutations in MSH2 and MLH1. *Journal of Medical Genetics* **37**, 641–645

Vasen HFA, Griffioen G, Offerhaus GJA *et al.* (1990). The value of screening and central registration of families with familial adenomatous polyposis. A study of 82 families in the Netherlands. *Diseases of the Colon and Rectum* **33**, 227–230

Vasen HF, Mecklin JP, Watson P *et al.* (1993). Surveillance in hereditary non polyposis colorectal cancer: an international study of 165 families. *Diseases of the Colon and Rectum* **36**, 1–4

Vasen HFA, van der Luijt RB, Slors JFM *et al.* (1996a). Molecular genetics tests as a guide to surgical management of familial adenomatous polyposis. *The Lancet* **348**, 433–435

Vasen HAS, Wijnen JT, Menko FH *et al.* (1996b) Cancer risk in families with hereditary non polyposis colorectal cancer diagnosed by mutation analysis. *Gastroenterology* **110**, 1020–1027

Vasen, Bulow SM, Myrhoj T *et al.* (1997) Decision analysis in the management of duodenal adenomatosis in familial adenomatous polyposis. *Gut* **40**, 716–719

Vasen HFA, van Ballegooijen M, Buskens E *et al.* (1998). A cost effectiveness analysis of colorectal screening of hereditary nonpolyposis colorectal carcinoma gene carriers. *Cancer* **82**, 1632–1637

Warthin AS (1913) Hereditary with reference to carcinoma. *Archives of Internal Medicine* **12**, 546–555

Weber T (1996) Clinical surveillance recommendations adopted for HNPCC. *The Lancet* **348**, 465

West Midlands Health Authority (1995). Cancer and health: Joint report of the West Midlands regional director of public health and the West Midlands regional cancer registry. *Uterine Cancer* 44–53

Woolf CM (1958). A genetic study of carcinoma of the large intestine. *American Journal of Human Genetics* **10**, 42–47

Chapter 4

Effectiveness of colorectal cancer screening

Wendy S Atkin

Introduction

There is no screening programme in the UK for colorectal cancer (CRC) despite the fact that the disease fulfils most of the criteria for screening stipulated by the World Health Organization (WHO: Wilson & Yungner 1968), with mortality rates higher than either breast or cervix cancer, for which there are screening programmes. CRC is the third most common cancer in both men and women and the second most frequent cause of cancer death in this country. The lifetime risk of developing the disease is 5% in both men and women, and it costs the NHS in excess of £200 million annually to treat (Dunlop 1997). Of the more than 30,000 new cases diagnosed each year, 60% die of the disease within 5 years. Yet when detected at an early, localised stage, 90% of cases can be cured and, when detected at the pre-malignant adenoma stage, cancer preventive treatment is virtually 100% effective (Atkin *et al.* 1992). Early cancers and adenomas are usually asymptomatic, so CRC would appear to be a good candidate for screening.

Two methods of screening for CRC have been intensively investigated: the faecal occult blood test (FOBT) and flexible sigmoidoscopy (FS). In the USA, screening as a method of reducing CRC mortality is now actively promoted, following the recommendation of the US Preventive Services Task Force (Levin & Bond 1996) that all men and women should undergo annual FOBT and periodic FS from age 50. This advice followed publication of the results of several randomised trials demonstrating a reduction in mortality after the use of FOBT (Mandel *et al.* 1993; Hardcastle *et al.* 1996; Kronborg *et al.* 1996) and of a case–control study (Selby *et al.* 1992) showing that screening sigmoidoscopy reduces the risk of development of CRC.

In the UK, there has been a more cautious approach to the adoption of CRC screening (Calman 1994). The importance of the disease and its suitability for screening and attention are now recognised, however, and attention is focused on investigating the extent to which each of the candidates for implementation in a national programme, FOBT and FS, is likely to be effective when offered outside the context of a research protocol. The aim of this review is to summarise what is known and what still needs to be learned before a decision is made about introducing CRC screening and which method to use.

Efficacy, effectiveness and efficiency

Before considering the specific properties of the CRC screening agents FOBT and FS, it is worth examining the terms used to describe the utility of interventions: efficacy, effectiveness and efficiency. These were first defined by a WHO Expert group in 1970 (White 2000) as follows.

Efficacy

The benefit or utility to the individual of the service, treatment regimen, drug, or preventive or control measure advocated or applied.

Effectiveness

The effect of the activity and the end-results, outcomes or benefits for the population achieved in relation to the stated objectives.

Efficiency

The effects or end-results achieved in relation to the effort expended in terms of money, resources and time.

Cochrane (1972) subsequently defined efficacy as the extent to which an intervention does more good than harm *under ideal circumstances* of healthcare practice whereas effectiveness assesses the same when provided under *usual circumstances* of healthcare practice.

The efficacy of a screening test for CRC is therefore a measure of the reduction in incidence or mortality from the disease *in those who use it, under ideal circumstances*. The effectiveness of a CRC screening test is a measure of the overall reduction in incidence or mortality *in the whole community offered the test*. A screening test is not usually used in isolation and it is therefore more usual to speak of the effectiveness of a screening programme. Thus, the effectiveness of a CRC screening programme will depend on the proportion of the population who use the test (not just on a single occasion in the case of a test that should be used at regular intervals for maximum efficacy). It will also depend on the diagnostic accuracy of the test and subsequent investigative procedures, and the safety and quality of endoscopic and surgical treatment that prevail in that community.

The sensitivity of a test is the proportion of cases detected by the test and affects efficacy. The specificity of a test is the proportion of individuals who do not have the disease and are correctly identified as negative. Its corollary, false positivity, is the proportion of negative individuals who test positive. False positivity can have a profound effect on efficiency in wasting resources in the investigation of those who do not have the disease.

Measuring efficacy and effectiveness

Most clinical trials attempt to measure efficacy. Clinical trials, however, are analysed on an intention-to-treat basis and, in population-based screening trials, the ability to measure efficacy is affected by uptake rates in the intervention group and exposure to screening in the control group (generally called contamination), e.g. if a screening test, applied under ideal circumstances, reduces incidence of CRC by 50%, but only 50% of the intervention group who are invited to use the test actually use it, the maximum difference in incidence that can be observed between the intervention and control groups as a whole is 25%. One way to overcome this problem is to undertake some form of pre-randomisation selection to reduce contamination of the groups by exclusion of those individuals who have already used the screening test, and including only those who state that they would use the test if they were offered it. This method has been used in a randomised trial of flexible sigmoidoscopy screening, described later. Some screening experts have criticised this methodology, arguing that trials should measure effectiveness because results from efficacy trials are not generalisable. An alternative view proposed by Haynes (1999) is that, if an intervention does not work under ideal conditions, there is little point in measuring it under less than ideal circumstances. Hawe (2000) supports this notion, stating that, if we are too ready to accept the real world conditions of effectiveness trials, we may risk a proliferation of state-of-the-art evaluations of less than state-of-the-art interventions.

Examining efficacy is, however, not sufficient: it is also important to understand how the test would perform in practice. The best model for estimating effectiveness appears to be the demonstration project or pilot. It is quite likely that the prevailing 'usual' circumstances in a pilot will leave much room for improvement. In the case of breast cancer screening, effectiveness has improved considerably since it was first introduced in a national screening programme: compliance rates have increased and the technology and diagnostic accuracy have also improved. One valuable aim of a demonstration project is to identify the resources required to raise the effectiveness of an intervention to approach that of the efficacy achieved in a trial, and to make a decision on whether the expenditure is worthwhile.

Faecal occult blood test

The theoretical basis for the FOBT is the assumption that asymptomatic, early stage, localised and therefore curable, cancers bleed, and that the small quantities of blood lost from the tumour can be detected in the stool. Blood lost in stool contains a mixture of intact haemoglobin, intact haem and its breakdown products. The most commonly used occult blood tests are guaiac based. Guaiac is a colourless gum that changes to a blue colour in the presence of haem or haemoglobin when developed with hydrogen peroxide. The most studied and widely available guaiac test is Haemoccult II. It has a low sensitivity for asymptomatic cancers (30–50%), but it has a high specificity of around 98%. As CRCs bleed intermittently, it is usual to recommend that two samples from each of three consecutive stools are collected and smeared on to six cards.

Results of FOBT trials

There have been three randomised trials of FOB screening that have reported their results. The two European trials (Hardcastle *et al*. 1996; Kronborg *et al*. 1996) have attempted to measure 'effectiveness' by inviting unselected members of the population, so that the reduction in mortality observed in the trials is likely to be achievable in a screening programme. The US trial undertaken in Minnesota (Mandel *et al*. 1993) was slightly different in that the participants were volunteers selected from the American Cancer Society, and veterans and employee groups. A total of 46,551 individuals aged 50–80 years were assigned to screening every year or every 2 years, or to a control group. False-positive or -negative results can occur with FOBT because of interference caused by components of the diet. In the Minnesota study, participants were instructed to refrain from red meat, poultry, fish and certain raw vegetables and fruit, and to stop taking vitamin C and aspirin for 24 hours before and during sample collection. It was noted that processing of the slides could be delayed by up to 8 days because of mailing delays and it was suspected that the resultant drying of the slides might decrease sensitivity. From 1977, therefore, the slides were rehydrated by adding a drop of water during processing. Participants with one or more of the six slides testing positive were evaluated initially by barium enema and later, when it was discovered that 20% of cancers were being missed by this method, this was replaced by colonoscopy. During follow-up, participants in all three groups were sent questionnaires or telephoned to assess their vital status. At 13 years it was found (Mandel *et al*. 1993) that the cumulative mortality in the annually screened group was 33% lower than in the control group. At this stage there was no significant reduction in mortality in the group offered 2-yearly screening and no reduction in incidence in either of the screened groups. By 18 years, the cumulative mortality in the biennial group was 21% lower than in the control group (Mandel *et al*. 1999) and it was noted (Mandel *et al*. 2000) that the cumulative incidence ratios were reduced by 20% and 17% for the annual and biennially screened groups, respectively, compared with the control group. It was concluded that the reduction in incidence resulted from the detection of large polyps by the FOBT that were subsequently removed at colonoscopy.

What factors might be expected to affect the generalisability of the results observed in the Minnesota trial? First, the compliance rates achieved were very high. The annual group completed 75% and the biennial group completed 78% of all screening tests offered. At least one test was completed by 90% of each group. Second, 82% of the FOBT slides were rehydrated, leading to an increase in sensitivity, but at the cost of a great increase in the positivity rate from 2.4% to 9.8%. As a result, by the time of first analysis at 13 years, 38% of the annual group and 28% of the biennial group had had at least one colonoscopy. The high rate of colonoscopy led Ransohoff and Lang (1990) to conclude that around a third to a half of the benefit of the FOBT screening was the result of the chance selection for colonoscopy caused, in turn, by the high positivity rate of FOBT for reasons other than a bleeding polyp or cancer.

The second trial (Hardcastle *et al.* 1996) was undertaken between 1981 and 1991 in Nottingham, England. A total of 152,850 people aged 45–74 years were randomly allocated to biennial screening with Haemoccult, or to a control group that was not offered screening. FOB tests were not rehydrated and dietary restriction was recommended only for re-testing borderline results. Individuals with either negative results or positive results but no neoplasia found at colonoscopy were invited to repeat the test every 2 years. At least one test was completed by 60% of the screening group and 38% completed all of the tests offered; 40% did not complete any test. The positivity rate was 2.1% after the first screen and 1.2% after any subsequent test and, by 14 years, there was a 15% reduction in CRC mortality.

The third trial (Kronborg *et al.* 1996) was undertaken in Denmark from 1985 onwards, using a protocol similar to that of the Nottingham study. A total of 137,485 people aged 45–75 were randomised to biennial screening or control groups. There was no rehydration of the slides but dietary restriction was recommended. Five rounds of screening were offered, and only those people who completed the first round were invited to undertake screening in subsequent rounds. The compliance rate in the first round was 67% and in subsequent rounds 92–94%. The positivity rate was around 1% at each of the rounds. By 10 years the cumulative CRC mortality was reduced by 18%. In neither the Nottingham nor the Danish trials has a reduction in incidence yet been observed.

The results of these trials suggest that offering FOBT screening reduces CRC mortality by 15–21% if offered every other year and by 33% if offered every year. However, it is unclear why the reduction in mortality in the biennially screened group in the US trial (20%) was similar to that in the European trials (15–18%), despite the higher compliance rates and the much higher positivity rates and overall exposure to colonoscopy resulting from the use of rehydration, which supposedly increased sensitivity.

Effectiveness of FOBT

What do the results of these research trials tell us about the likely effectiveness of a national programme? First, to be effective, compliance rates have to be relatively high. It is particularly important that rates are high at older ages because CRC incidence rates increase exponentially with age. A fall-off in compliance with repeated testing has been noted in several community-based FOBT screening programmes (Neilson & Whynes 1995; Wei *et al.* 1998). If screening is started at age 50 when CRC rates are low, compliance may have decreased to unacceptably low levels by the late 60s when the test will have been offered several times. Apart from low socioeconomic status, which is associated with low rates of participation in virtually all health interventions, factors specific to decreased compliance with FOBT include male sex, the requirement for dietary restriction, an absence of symptoms, not wanting to know about health problems and the technical difficulties with the test (Farrands *et al.* 1984; Macrae *et al.* 1984; Hart *et al.* 1998).

Failure to investigate screen positives is another problem with the FOBT. A recent study from the USA found that only a third of screen positives underwent colonic evaluation (Lurie & Welch 1999). If this is common practice, population screening is likely to be more costly and less effective in the USA than estimated from controlled trials. In the Danish trial, 85% of screen positives underwent colonoscopy, suggesting that FOBT should be offered only as part of an organised programme.

UK pilot of FOBT screening

In the UK, there is a clear framework for the initiation of new screening programmes in the NHS (Calman 1994). After the publication of the results of the randomised trials from the UK and Denmark, the National Screening Committee held two workshops to assess the feasibility of CRC screening by FOBT. It was concluded that a demonstration pilot project was required to examine whether implementing biennial FOBT as part of a national screening programme within the NHS will reduce mortality at reasonable cost and without undue morbidity (http://www.doh.gov.uk/nsc/pdfs/summary). A pilot study was started in 2000 and will last for 2 years. It includes two centres: Fife, Grampian and Tayside in Scotland (1.2 million population) and Coventry and Warwick in England (800,000 population). The age group invited is 50–69 years and one half of this age group are being offered the test in the first year and the other half in the second year.

The pilot studies have been set up as would be necessary in a programme and the organisation is complex. An information system was developed for identification of eligible individuals, invitation of these individuals for screening, controlling and monitoring their progress through the screening process, recording test results and results of subsequent investigations and treatment, and the production of performance statistics for the formal independent evaluation. There is a central office and laboratory in each of the two sites with responsibility for mailing tests, receiving and processing completed tests, mailing test results, and organising repeat tests and colonoscopies for FOBT positives. A telephone helpline is available at each site to answer queries and, it is hoped, to prevent test recipients from seeking advice from their general practitioner, and several specialist nurses have been employed to explain a positive test (the necessity for a colonoscopy), and the need for re-testing in the case of equivocal results. Each centre has drawn up common protocols and quality assurance standards for all procedures. The expert organisation results from years of experience in the UK in the implementation of the breast and cervical cancer screening programmes. At the end of the 2-year period, the results collected by the independent evaluation group will be analysed and decisions made about whether to continue to offer the test to the population and whether to implement it more widely in a screening programme within the NHS.

Flexible sigmoidoscopy

The 60-cm flexible sigmoidoscope is a short version of the colonoscope that can be used to examine the sigmoid colon and rectum, where 60% of CRCs and adenomas are located. FS has a number of advantages over FOBT as a screening agent. It is highly sensitive for the detection of adenomas so that FS screening may be more efficacious in reducing CRC incidence rates. In addition, most adenomas can be removed during the screening procedure, avoiding the anxiety associated with a positive test. Third, the progression of an adenomatous polyp to cancer is a slow process taking 10 years or more (Winawer *et al.* 1987), so targeting the adenoma rather than cancer in screening for CRC means that, at least theoretically, the test can be undertaken less frequently. Although FS screening intervals of 3–5 years are recommended in the USA, the protection afforded by a single FS may last for up to 10 years (Selby *et al.* 1992) or even longer, depending on the age at which it is undertaken (Atkin *et al.* 1993). The duration of protection of a single FS is being examined as part of the UK randomised trial of once-only FS screening.

Compliance with FS screening

Compliance with FS screening is highly variable, with rates as high as 95% among US Government personnel (Wherry & Thomas 1994) and as low as 12% among 55- to 59-year-old Australian citizens chosen at random from the electoral register (Olynyk *et al.* 1996). In two UK population-based studies, attendance for screening was 45% and 49%, respectively (Atkin *et al.* 1998; Verne *et al.* 1998). Factors affecting compliance with FS screening are similar to those with FOBT screening, although attendance rates are higher in men than in women whereas the converse is true with FOBT (Faivre *et al.* 1991; Herold *et al.* 1997; Wei *et al.* 1998).

Preventing proximal colon cancer

A major disadvantage of FS is that the proximal colon, where about 40% of adenomas and cancers are located, is not examined. Some proximal lesions can be detected by undertaking colonoscopy in those with a distal adenoma, because distal adenomas are associated with a two- to threefold increased risk of having proximal adenomas (Collett *et al.* 1999). Most proximal adenomas, however, do not progress to cancer and the risks of their removal may outweigh the possible benefit. Advanced adenomas have a higher malignant potential and may be a more suitable target for screening in the less accessible proximal colon. Several studies suggest that the risk of having an advanced adenoma (large, villous, severely dysplastic) or cancer in the proximal colon is related to the characteristics of distal adenomas (Atkin *et al.* 1992; Zarchy & Ershoff 1994). There is a three- to fourfold increased risk of colon cancer in those with a large or villous distal adenoma, but there is no increased risk in those with only small tubular adenomas. The risks and costs of colonoscopy are probably warranted only in the 5% of people found at FS screening to have high-risk adenomas (Atkin *et al.* 1993).

Undertaking colonoscopy in those with adenomas for the purpose of preventing proximal cancer is bound to be largely ineffective because 75% of cases of proximal colon cancer occur without an index lesion in the distal colon (Lemmel *et al.* 1996). This has led to calls in the USA (Podolsky 2000) for colonoscopy screening. Advantages are the ability to detect, at a single examination, both proximal and distal lesions. The disadvantages are that it is invasive, expensive and inconvenient, involving at least 36 hours of commitment in preparing the bowel and recovering from the sedation given routinely during the procedure. By contrast, FS requires no sedation, and bowel preparation involves only a single enema that can be self-administered at home (Atkin *et al.* 2000). Acceptance rates with colonoscopy are low (Rex *et al.* 1993; Lieberman *et al.* 2000) and complication rates (haemorrhage and perforation) are higher than for FS (Waye *et al.* 1996). Furthermore, there is no evidence that colonoscopy is more efficacious than FS, and in two studies (Muller & Sonnenberg 1995; Kavanagh *et al.* 1998), no additional benefit was observed in terms of reduction in incidence of CRC after colonoscopy compared with FS.

Published evidence on efficacy of FS screening

Several epidemiological studies have shown that after (mostly rigid) sigmoidoscopy there is a 60–80% decreased incidence of distal bowel cancer (Gilbertsen & Nelms 1978; Newcomb *et al.* 1992; Selby *et al.* 1992; Muller & Sonnenberg 1995) suggesting that the detection and removal of adenomatous polyps reduces incidence of CRC. However, only two randomised controlled trials have been published (Friedman *et al.* 1986; Thiis-Evensen *et al.* 1999), both of which were too small to demonstrate a beneficial effect of adenoma removal. The most influential of the remaining studies is a case–control study (Selby *et al.* 1992) undertaken using the records kept by the Kaiser Permanente Health Maintenance Organisation (HMO). This study compared the exposure to sigmoidoscopy screening during the previous 10 years of cases with a diagnosis of fatal distal CRC and age- and sex-matched controls. The risk of developing distal CRC was reduced by 60% in those undergoing sigmoidoscopy screening. The possibility that the effect was the result of selection bias was reduced by the observation that sigmoidoscopy had no effect on reducing incidence of cancer in the proximal colon beyond the reach of the sigmoidoscope.

There is some evidence that sigmoidoscopic screening may be having an impact on CRC incidence rates in the USA. A recent analysis (Rabeneck *et al.* 2001) of the temporal changes in incidence was undertaken using data held by Registries of the Surveillance, Epidemiology and End Results (SEER) which covers 14% of the US population. A decrease in CRC incidence rates between 1989 and 1997 was demonstrated for distal colon cancer in white men and women, and to a lesser extent in black men and women. During this period there was no change in proximal colon cancer rates. The US Centers for Disease Control (CDC) recently published the results (CDC 2001) of a survey undertaken in 1999 in 50 states among people aged

≥ 50 years, which showed that on average 20.6% of the population had had an FOBT during the previous year and 33.6% had had a sigmoidoscopy or colonoscopy within the previous 5 years. Although these rates are regarded as low in the USA, where there are national guidelines recommending FOBT and sigmoidoscopic screening, it is possibly high enough to account for the declines in distal CRC incidence rates.

On-going trials of FS screening

In the UK, the randomised trial is still considered the gold standard and a requirement for consideration of a screening modality for a national screening programme. Three randomised trials of FS screening are in progress: the PLCO (prostate, lung, colon, ovary) trial in the USA is examining the efficacy of 5-yearly FS screening, whereas trials in the UK and in Italy are evaluating the effect of a single FS screen offered at age 55–64 years. These are described below.

The PLCO trial (Prorok *et al.* 2000) is a US trial sponsored by the National Cancer Institute which is examining the effect of colon and prostate cancer screening in men and colon and ovarian cancer screening in women; both male and female smokers are being offered lung cancer screening. This multicentre trial, which began in 1994, aims to randomise 148,000 people (equal numbers of men and women) (Simpson *et al.* 2000). Recruitment is almost complete and approximately half the cohort has been offered a second round of screening. Further details may be found on the NCI website (http://dcp.nci.nih.gov/plco/).

The UK trial (Atkin *et al.* 2001) is evaluating the efficacy and acceptability of a screening regimen, which includes:

- a single FS screen at age 55–64 years, with
- removal of all small adenomas during FS, and
- colonoscopy only for those found to have 'high-risk' polyps, which includes any of the following: multiple (≥ 3), large (≥ 1 cm), tubulovillous, villous or severely dysplastic adenomas or those with more than 20 hyperplastic polyps above the distal rectum.

The Italian trial (Senore *et al.* 1996; Segnan *et al.* 1999) is using the UK protocol with a few small modifications, including the stipulation in the criteria for colonoscopy that all polyps larger than 5 mm are should be considered 'high risk' irrespective of histopathology.

There are 14 UK trial centres and six Italian centres. The UK trial includes patients of designated GPs who were not excluded by their GP because of a terminal disease, a history of CRC or adenomas, inflammatory bowel disease or recent screening, or were unable to provide informed consent. General practices were selected in order to produce a mix of small and large practices and a good spread across the catchment area of the hospital in each centre. The trial used a two-stage recruitment procedure to reduce contamination between the groups, which arises when participants in the control group gain access to screening and those in the intervention group fail to undergo screening. At the first stage of recruitment, potentially eligible individuals were sent an 'interest in screening' questionnaire, and those who expressed an interest in having the screening test and did not meet the exclusion criteria were randomised to the intervention or control groups. The intervention group was then invited for FS screening whereas the control group was not contacted.

Recruitment and screening in both the UK and the Italian trials are now complete. In the UK 368,597 people were sent 'interest in screening' questionnaires, of whom 53% expressed interest in having screening by FS. Of the 57,070 randomised to the intervention group and invited for screening, 71% attended. At FS screening, the detection rates of polyps, adenomas and cancers were 25, 12 and 0.3%, respectively. As predicted, 5% of people undergoing screening required a colonoscopy because of the detection at FS of 'high-risk' adenomas. Cancer was detected in 140 cases, 62% of which were localised cases (24 were removed endoscopically and 63 were surgically removed Dukes' A stage cases). There were five perforations, equating to only one in over 40,000 FS and 4 in 2,377 colonoscopies (0.17%). The perforation rate at colonoscopy is similar to other published rates (Waye *et al.* 1996). The low rate of perforations at FS is also similar to reported rates (Anderson *et al.* 2000), but is remarkable in the FS screening study because over 10,000 polyps were removed during screening. There have been four procedure-related deaths, all following surgery.

All participants in the trial are being followed up using records held by the Office of National Statistics (ONS). The end-points of the study are diagnosis of and death from CRC. As a result of the need not to delay the analysis of outcome, it is likely that the records of local cancer registries will be used in addition to those held at ONS and that intermediate end-points will be used in the first instance.

In the Italian trial (Segnan *et al.* 1999), only 18% (33,448 people) responded positively to the mailed 'interest in screening' questionnaire. Among the 17,164 randomised to the intervention group, however, 58% have attended. In the Italian protocol, colonoscopy was indicated for all polyps larger than 6 mm and, as a result, 8.6% underwent colonoscopy compared with 5% in the UK trial.

Preparing for a national screening programme in the UK

Three clinical trials have demonstrated that CRC screening by FOBT would have a modest reduction in mortality rates. Trials are on-going to test the hypothesis that screening for and removing distal colorectal adenomas would reduce incidence rates. The 40% attendance rates achieved in the UK FS screening trial, which can be considered high in the absence of media and health educational promotion, and the high rates of compliance with FOBT achieved in the Nottingham trial, suggest that the UK population want CRC screening.

The Department of Health has shown its commitment to CRC screening by undertaking a pilot study of FOBT, the result of which will be analysed by 2003. Thus, it appears that the crucial decision about whether to implement a CRC screening programme and which method to use will be made within the next 2 years.

The challenge will be to provide the means to deliver a high-quality programme. One difficulty that can be anticipated is the chronic shortage of endoscopy resources, including trained medical or nurse endoscopists, support staff and equipment. A recent British Society of Gastroenterology audit (Bowles *et al.* 2001) has reported that the expertise and training of current endoscopists leave much to be desired. In addition there are long waiting lists for colonoscopy for investigation of symptomatic patients. The under-investment in endoscopy services may well be, at least partially, responsible for the low survival rates from CRC in the UK compared with other countries (Evans & Pritchard 2000; Gatta *et al.* 2000). If the UK is to be in a position to introduce CRC, this problem needs to be addressed as a matter of urgency. The Director of Cancer Services, Professor Mike Richards, has committed £2.5 million over 3 years to pilot a training programme. This is a gross under-estimate of the amount required to rectify years of under-investment in gastrointestinal endoscopy, the most powerful tool currently available for CRC prevention.

References

Anderson M, Pasha T, Leighton J *et al.* (2000). Endoscopic perforation of the colon: lessons from a 10-year study. *American Journal of Gastroenterology* **95**, 3418–3422

Atkin WS, Morson BC, Cuzick J *et al.* (1992a). Long-term risk of colorectal cancer after excision of rectosigmoid adenomas [see comments]. *New England Journal of Medicine* **326**, 658–662

Atkin WS, Williams CB, Macrae FA, Jones S (1992b). Randomised study of surveillance intervals after removal of colorectal adenomas at colonoscopy. *Gut* **33**, S52

Atkin WS, Cuzick J, Northover JMA, Whyner DK (1993). Prevention of colorectal cancer by once-only sigmoidoscopy. *The Lancet* **341**, 736–740

Atkin WS, Hart A, Edwards R *et al.* (1998). Uptake, yield of neoplasia and adverse effects of flexible sigmoidoscopy. *Gut* **42**, 560–565

Atkin W, Hart A, Edwards R *et al.* (2000). Single-blind, randomised trial of the efficacy and acceptability of oral Picolax vs self-administered phosphate enema in bowel preparation for flexible sigmoidoscopy screening. *British Medical Journal* **320**, 1504–9

Atkin W, Edwards R, Wardle J *et al.* (2001). Rationale and design of a multicentre randomised trial to evaluate the suitability of flexible sigmoidoscopy as a mass population screening tool to reduce colorectal cancer morbidity and mortality. *Journal of Medical Screening* in press

Bowles C, Leicester R, Swarbrick E *et al.* (2001). Intercollegiate national-BSG colonoscopy (IBNC) audit: identification and management of polyps diagnosed at colonoscopy. *Gut* **48**(suppl 1), A10

Calman K (1994). Developing screening in the NHS. *Journal of Medical Screening* **2**, 101–104

Centers for Disease Control (2001). Trends in screening for colorectal cancer – United States, 1997 and 1999. *MMWR, Morbidity and Mortality Weekly Report* **50**, 162–166

Cochrane A (1972). *Effectiveness and Efficiency: Random reflections on health services.* London: Nuffield Provincial Hospitals Trust

Collett J, Platell C, Fletcher D, Aquila S, Olynyk J (1999). Distal colonic neoplasms predict proximal neoplasia in average-risk, asymptomatic subjects. *Journal of Gastroenterology and Hepatology* **14**, 67–71

Dunlop M (1997). Science, medicine, and the future – colorectal cancer. *British Medical Journal* **314**, 1882–1885

Evans B & Pritchard C (2000). Cancer survival rates and GDP expenditure on health: a comparison of England and Wales and the USA, Denmark, Netherlands, Finland, France, Germany, Italy, Spain and Switzerland in the 1990s. *Public Health* **114**, 336–339

Faivre J, Arveux P, Milan C *et al.* (1991). Participation in mass screening for colorectal cancer: results of screening and rescreening from the Burgundy study. *European Journal of Cancer Prevention* **1**, 49–55

Farrands PA, Hardcastle JD, Chamberlain J, Moss S (1984). Factors affecting compliance with screening for colorectal cancer. *Community Medicine* 12-1

Friedman GD, Collen MF, Fireman BH (1986). Multiphasic Health Checkup Evaluation: a 16-year follow-up. *Journal of Chronic Disease* **39**, 453–463

Gatta G, Capocaccia R, Sant M *et al.* (2000). Understanding variations in survival for colorectal cancer in Europe: a EUROCARE high resolution study. *Gut* **47**, 533–538

General Register Office, Scotland (1998) *Annual Report*

Gilbertsen VA & Nelms JM (1978). The prevention of invasive cancer of the rectum. *Cancer* **41**, 1137–1139

Hardcastle J, Chamberlain J, Robinson M *et al.* (1996). Randomised controlled trial of faecal-occult-blood screening for colorectal cancer. *The Lancet* **348**, 1472–1477

Hart A, Eaden J, Barnett S, Debono A, Mayberry J (1998). Colorectal-cancer prevention – an approach to increasing compliance in a fecal occult blood-test screening-program. *Journal of Epidemiology and Community Health* **52**, 818–820

Hawe P (2000). How much trial and error should we tolerate in community trials? (Letter to Editor). *British Medical Journal* **320**, 120

Haynes B (1999). Can it work? Does it work? Is it worth it? (Editorial). *British Medical Journal* **319**, 652–653

Herold A, Riker A, Warner E *et al.* (1997). Evidence of gender bias in patients undergoing flexible sigmoidoscopy. *Cancer Detection and Prevention* **21**, 141–147

Kavanagh A, Giovannucci E, Fuchs C, Colditz G (1998). Screening endoscopy and risk of colorectal cancer in united states men. *Cancer Causes and Control* **9**, 455–462

Kronborg O, Fenger C, Olsen J *et al.* (1996). Randomised study of screening for colorectal cancer with faecal-occult-blood test. *The Lancet* **348**, 1467–1471

Lemmel G, Haseman J, Rex D, Rahmani E (1996). Neoplasia distal to the splenic flexure in patients with proximal colon cancer. *Gastrointestinal Endoscopy* **44**, 109–111

Levin B & Bond J (1996). Colorectal cancer screening. Recommendations of the U.S. Preventive Services Task Force. *Gastroenterology* **111**, 1381–1384

Lieberman D, Weiss D, Bond J *et al.* (2000). Use of colonoscopy to screen asymptomatic adults for colorectal cancer. *New England Journal of Medicine* **343**, 162–168

Lurie J & Welch H (1999). Diagnostic testing following fecal occult blood screening in the elderly. *Journal of the National Cancer Institute* **91**, 1641

Macrae FA, Hill DJ, St John JB *et al.* (1984). Predicting colon cancer screening behaviour from health beliefs. *Preventive Medicine* **13**, 115–126

Mandel J, Bond J, Church T *et al.* (1993). Reducing mortality from colorectal cancer by screening for fecal occult blood. *New England Journal of Medicine* **328**, 1365–1371

Mandel J, Church T, Ederer F, Bond J (1999). Colorectal cancer mortality: Effectiveness of biennial screening for fecal occult blood. *Journal of the National Cancer Institute* **91**, 434–437

Mandel J, Church T, Bond J *et al.* (2000). The effect of fecal occult blood screening on the incidence of colorectal cancer. *New England Journal of Medicine* **343**, 1603–1607

Muller A & Sonnenberg A (1995). Prevention of colorectal cancer by flexible endoscopy and polypectomy. *Annals of Internal Medicine* **123**, 904–910

Neilson A & Whynes D (1995). Determinants of persistent compliance with screening for colorectal cancer. *Social Science and Medicine* **41**, 365–374

Newcomb PA, Norfleet RG, Storer B, Surawicz S, Marcus PM (1992). Screening sigmoidoscopy and colorectal cancer mortality. *Journal of the National Cancer Institute* **84**, 1572–1575

Northern Ireland Cancer Registry. Cancer Incidence data 1993–96 and mortality data 1993–98.

Office for National Statistics (1998). *Mortality Statistics*, Series DH2 no 25

Office for National Statistics (2000). *Health Statistics Quarterly* 6, Summer 2000

Olynyk J, Aquilia S, Fletcher D, Dickinson J (1996). Flexible sigmoidoscopy screening for colorectal-cancer in average-risk subjects – a community-based pilot project. *Medical Journal of Australia* **165**(2), 74–76

Podolsky D (2000). Going the distance – the case for true colorectal-cancer screening. *New England Journal of Medicine* **343**, 207–208

Prorok P, Andriole G, Bresalier R *et al.* (2000). Design of the Prostate, Lung, Colorectal and Ovarian (PLCO) Cancer Screening Trial. *Controlled Clinical Trials* **21**(suppl 6), 273S–309S

Rabeneck L, El-Serag H, Sandler R (2001). Incidence and survival of colorectal cancer in the US: 1989–1997. *Gastroenterology* **120**(suppl 1), A65

Ransohoff D & Lang C (1990). Small adenomas detected during fecal occult blood screening for colorectal cancer: the impact of serendipity. *Journal of the American Medical Association* **264**, 76–78

Rex D, Lehman G, Ulbright T *et al.* (1993). Colonic neoplasia in asymptomatic persons with negative fecal occult blood tests: influence of age, gender, and family history. *American Journal of Gastroenterology* **88**, 825–831

Scottish Cancer Intelligence Unit (1999). *Scottish Health Statistics*. Scotland: ISD

Segnan N, Sciallero S, Bonelli L *et al.* (1999). Multicentre randomised controlled trial of once only flexible sigmoidoscopy screening in Italy – score. *Endoscopy* **31**(suppl 1), E9

Selby JV, Friedman GD, Quesenberry CJ, Weiss NS (1992). A case-control study of screening sigmoidoscopy and mortality from colorectal cancer. *New England Journal of Medicine* **326**, 653–657

Senore C, Segnan N, Rossini F *et al.* (1996). Screening for colorectal cancer by once only sigmoidoscopy: a feasibility study in Turin, Italy. *Journal of Medical Screening* **3**, 72–78

Simpson N, Johnson C, Ogden S *et al.* (2000). Recruitment strategies in the Prostate, Lung, Colorectal and Ovarian (PLCO) Cancer Screening Trial: The first six years. *Controlled Clinical Trials* **21**(suppl 6), 356S–378S

Thiis-Evensen E, Hoff G, Sauar J *et al.* (1999). Population-based surveillance by colonoscopy: effect on the incidence of colorectal cancer. Telemark Polyp Study I. *Scandinavian Journal of Gastroenterology* **34**, 414–420

Verne J, Aubrey R, Love S, Talbot I, Northover J (1998). Population based randomised study of uptake and yield of screening by flexible sigmoidoscopy compared with screening by faecal occult blood testing. *British Medical Journal* **317**, 182–185

Waye J, Kahn O, Auerbach M (1996). Complications of colonoscopy and flexible sigmoidoscopy. *Gastrointestinal Endoscopic Clinics of North America* **6**, 343–377

Wei N, Nakama H, Li T (1998). Screen compliance rates in 14-years annual screening program for colorectal cancer with immunochemical fecal occult blood test – identification of higher priority subjects in health education. *European Journal of Medical Research* **3**, 341–344

Wherry DC & Thomas WM (1994). The yield of flexible fiberoptic sigmoidoscopy in the detection of asymptomatic colorectal neoplasia. *Surgical Endoscopy* **8**, 393–395

White K (2000). Cochrane may not have been the first to define efficacy and effectiveness. *British Medical Journal* **320**, 121

Wilson JMG & Yungner G (1968). *The Principles and Practice of Screening for Disease.* Geneva: WHO

Winawer S, Zauber AG, Diaz B, Workgroup NPS (1987). The National Polyp Study: temporal sequence of evolving colorectal cancer from normal mucosa. *Gastrointestinal Endoscopy* **33**, 167

Zarchy TM & Ershoff D (1994). Do characteristics of adenomas on flexible sigmoidoscopy predict advanced lesions on baseline colonoscopy? *Gastroenterology* **106**, 1501–1504

PART 2

Evidence and opinion for medical intervention

Chapter 5

Scientific evidence and expert clinical opinion for adjuvant chemotherapy after curatively resected colon cancer

Nick Maisey and Mark Hill

Introduction

The role of adjuvant chemotherapy after curatively resected node-positive colon cancer is now well established. Controversies remain, however, surrounding the optimal chemotherapy regimen, whether to treat node-negative patients and other issues of patient selection. This chapter examines the evidence regarding these questions, and explores the introduction of novel agents in this setting.

A number of large prospective randomised trials have now beyond doubt recognised the value of 5-fluorouracil (5FU)-based chemotherapy in the adjuvant treatment of stage III (Dukes' C) colon cancer (Table 5.1). The first of these was the National Surgical Adjuvant Breast and Bowel Project (NSABP) C-01 trial (Wolmark *et al.* 1988). In this study 1,166 patients with resected Dukes' B and C colorectal cancer were randomised among surgery alone, BCG (Bacille Calmette–Guérin) and MOF chemotherapy (methyl-lomustine, vincristine and bolus 5FU 325 mg/m^2). BCG had no effect on outcome compared with surgery alone, whereas the MOF regimen resulted in a 24% reduction in the risk of death ($p = 0.05$), improving overall survival rate at 5 years from 59% to 67% ($p = 0.05$). In the three-arm Intergroup study, 1,296 patients with resected Dukes' B and C tumours were randomised among surgery alone, levamisole and bolus 5FU with levamisole (Moertel *et al.* 1990). The updated results confirm that, with a median follow-up of 6.5 years, the 5FU arm reduced the risk of death by 33% ($p < 0.0007$) (Moertel *et al.* 1995). O'Connell *et al.* (1997) demonstrated an advantage for the eponymous 5FU-based Northern Central Cancer Treatment Group (NCCTG) regimen over surgery alone in patients with Dukes' B and C tumours. This regimen reduced the risk of death by 16% ($p = 0.02$) and improved overall survival from 63% to 74% compared with surgery alone. Finally, the IMPACT (International Multicentre Pooled Analysis of Colon Cancer Trials) study analysed pooled data from four relatively small studies comparing bolus 5FU regimens with surgery alone (Anonymous 1995). Overall use of 5FU-based chemotherapy was associated with a reduction in the risk of death of 22%.

Table 5.1 Pivotal studies of adjuvant chemotherapy versus surgery alone in Dukes' C colorectal cancer

Study	n	Dukes' stage	Chemotherapy	Reduction in risk of death (%)	p
NSABP C-01 (Wolmark et al. 1988)	1,166	B + C	MOF	26	0.05
Intergroup (Moertal et al. 1995)	929	C	5FU + Lev	33	0.007
NCCTG (O'Connell et al. 1997)	317	B + C	5FU + FA	16	0.02
IMPACT (Anonymous 1995)	1,526	B + C	5FU + FA	22	0.029

MOF, methyl-lomustine (methyl-CCNU), vincristine (Oncovin) and bolus 5FU; Lev, levamisole; FA, folinic acid.

Controversies in adjuvant chemotherapy for colon cancer

Although there is no doubt that chemotherapy should be offered to fit patients with resected Dukes' C tumours, there is debate over the value of such intervention in those with Dukes' B2 tumours. The optimal schedule of administration and duration of 5FU-based chemotherapy remains controversial and recently published data have provided new insights (Saini et al. 2000). Advances in molecular biology have revealed a number of potential prognostic markers which may refine our treatment algorithms, but which require confirmation in large prospective studies. The introduction of a number of novel agents has added to our armamentarium in advanced disease and these are currently being evaluated in randomised trials in an adjuvant setting. The role of preoperative radiotherapy in locally advanced tumours and the therapeutic ratio of adjuvant treatment in elderly and/or medically unfit patients also require further elucidation.

Adjuvant chemotherapy in Dukes' B2 tumours

The debate surrounding the use of adjuvant chemotherapy in Dukes' B2 tumours has been confounded by a number of factors. The relatively favourable results of surgery alone in these patients mean that any advantage conferred by the addition of chemotherapy is likely to be small, and therefore a large number of patients would be required to detect such a difference. The randomised studies of adjuvant chemotherapy have often had only a small subgroup of B2 tumours, the majority being Dukes' C histology, and so they are often statistically underpowered (Table 5.2). The use of a variety of chemotherapy regimens has also confused the issue.

Table 5.2 Pivotal studies of adjuvant chemotherapy in Dukes' B tumours

Intergroup Study (Moertel *et al.* 1995; *n* = 325)

Treatment	7-year disease-free survival rate (%)	Yearly overall survival rate (%)
Surgery alone	71	72
Surgery + 5FU/Lev	79	72
p	0.1	NS

NSABP Study (Mamounas *et al.* 1999; *n* = 1,567)

Trial	Treatment	Overall survival rate (%)	p
C-01	Surgery	72	0.73
	MOF	75	
C-02	Surgery	76	0.005
	PVI-5FU	78	
C-03	MOF	84	0.03
	5FU/FA	92	
C-04	5FU/Lev	81	0.25
	5FU/FA	85	

IMPACT-B2 (Anonymous 1999; *n* = 1,016)

Treatment	5-year event-free survival rate (%)	5-year overall survival rate (%)
5FU/FA	76	82
Surgery alone	73	80
p	NS	NS

In the Intergroup study, 325 patients with B2 tumours were included. Patients were randomised between surgery alone and surgery followed by 5FU and levamisole (Moertel *et al.* 1995). Although there was no difference in overall survival after 7 years of follow-up, there was a 32% reduction in recurrence rate in the treatment arm, similar to the reduction seen in the Dukes' C cohort. The disease-free survival rate was 79% and 71% (*p* = 0.1) for the chemotherapy arm and surgery-alone arm, respectively. A combined analysis of 1,567 patients with stage II tumours from four adjuvant NSABP studies also reported an advantage for adjuvant chemotherapy (Mamounas *et al.* 1999). A decrease in mortality and recurrence rate and an improvement in disease-free survival were noted irrespective of stage. Somewhat paradoxically, the reduction in mortality was higher for low-risk rather than high-risk Dukes' B tumours (32% vs 20%), although this may merely reflect the reduced efficacy of chemotherapy in more aggressive disease. Data from five trials were pooled and analysed in the IMPACT B2 study (Anonymous 1999). Over 1,000 patients (*n* = 1,016) with node-negative tumours were analysed, and the results at first sight appear to contradict the data from the NSABP analysis. There was no significant difference in both 5-year event-free survival rates (76% vs 73%) and overall survival rates (82% vs 80%) in the adjuvant and surgery-alone arm, respectively. However, it must be noted that the dose of 5FU ranged between 370 and 425 mg/m^2 in the five trials studied, with a majority at the lower end of the dose range. If total dose delivered or dose intensity is important in this setting, as seems likely, then the differences in outcome may not be so difficult to explain.

Thus, although there is evidence to support the use of adjuvant chemotherapy in Dukes' B2 tumours, proof beyond doubt is still lacking. Having reviewed the available evidence in detail, many centres, including our own, have concluded that there is a good case for offering treatment to fit patients in this category. Two large well-conducted studies (the Intergroup study and the NSABP study) both demonstrate a reduction in the risk of death that is similar to that of stage III cancers (around 30%). Although the IMPACT B2 study did not corroborate this finding, many patients were arguably under-treated. There is an urgent need for further research in this area. Until further data are available, we feel that a pragmatic individualised approach is justified, where the benefits of chemotherapy and potential toxicities are discussed at length with patients, and a joint, fully informed decision is reached. The situation is somewhat different in older patients and those with less good performance status or other medical problems, where a more conservative approach is usually recommended.

What is the optimal 5FU-based chemotherapy regimen?

It is generally accepted that the current 'gold standard' regimen for adjuvant chemotherapy is a combination of 5FU and folinic acid, administered as bolus treatment for a period of 6 months. Folinic acid increases and prolongs the inhibition of thymidylate synthase, the target enzyme of 5FU. Its combination with 5FU has been shown conclusively to improve disease-free survival and overall survival compared with modulation by levamisole, with a 25–30% decrease in the odds of dying from colon cancer (O'Connell *et al.* 1998; Wolmark *et al.* 1999). The study by O'Connell *et al.* (1998) randomised patients to receive either folinic acid or levamisole to modulate 5FU, with a second randomisation to either 6 or 12 months of treatment. This study demonstrated that the shorter duration of treatment did not appear to have any detrimental effects on survival.

Data from our institution published in the last year have taken this argument further (Saini *et al.* 2000). The use of protracted venous infused (PVI) 5FU has been shown to be associated with higher response rates (Table 5.3) and lower toxicity (Table 5.4) in patients with metastatic disease (Anonymous 1998). The incidence of life-threatening toxicity, particularly haematological toxicity, is an important consideration in the design of an adjuvant regimen, particularly where the survival benefit is small. The reduced incidence of significant haematological toxicity associated with PVI-5FU favours its use over bolus schedules in this setting. A multi-centre study (SAFFA) instigated at the Royal Marsden Hospital was designed to examine the hypothesis that the improved therapeutic index of infused 5FU might enhance the eradication of micrometastatic disease in the adjuvant setting. After curative surgery for Dukes' B or C colorectal cancer, 697 patients were randomised to receive one of two regimens: either 24 weeks of the standard Mayo/NCCTG (bolus 5FU 425 mg/m^2 and folinic acid 20 mg/m^2 for 5 days on a 28-day cycle), or 12 weeks of PVI-5FU 300 mg/m^2. The two groups were well balanced in terms of baseline demographics and prognostic factors.

Table 5.3 Meta-analysis of response following PVI or bolus 5FU

Treatment modality	Complete response	Partial response	Overall response	Median response duration (months) (95%CI)
PVI	3	19	22	7.1 (5.7–8.5)
Bolus	2	12	14	6.7 (5.7–8.5)

Anonymous (1998).
Overall response odds ratio = 0.55; 95%CI, 0.41–0.75; p = 0.0002.

Table 5.4 Meta-analysis of common toxicities following PVI or bolus 5FU

Toxicity	PVI-5FU (%)	Bolus 5FU (%)	Adjusted RR	95%CI	p
Grade III–IV haematological	4	31	0.14	0.09–0.21	<0.0001
Grade III–IV non-haematological	13	14	0.96	0.72–1.28	0.78
Diarrhoea	4	6			
Nausea/Vomiting	3	4			
Mucositis	9	7			
Hand–foot syndrome	34	13	1.87	1.50–2.34	< 0.0001

Anonymous (1998).
RR, risk ratio (PVI: bolus); CI, confidence interval.

Analysis of grade III–IV toxicity revealed a significant reduction in diarrhoea, stomatitis, alopecia and neutropenia in the PVI-5FU arm (Table 5.5). Only 8% of patients required Hickman line replacement. Global quality of life (measured by the EORTC QLQ-C30 questionnaire) was significantly inferior on the bolus 5FU arm within the first 4 weeks of treatment (p = 0.019) (Figure 5.1), and returned to pre-treatment levels approximately 3 months later than the PVI-5FU arm (Figure 5.2). There was a significant improvement in relapse-free survival (p = 0.015) (Figure 5.3), although there was no detectable difference in overall survival between arms. There was a suggestion of an advantage in overall survival for the subgroup of patients with rectal tumours treated with the infused regimen (p = 0.07) (Figure 5.4).

It appears therefore that PVI-5FU is at least as effective as the bolus regimen, but importantly it is less toxic and has less of an impact on patients' quality of life. Recruitment is ongoing for patients with rectal tumours, and results are awaited with anticipation.

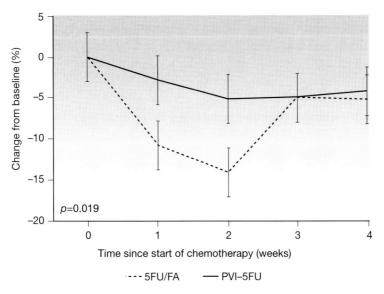

Figure 5.1 Change in global quality of life in the first 4 weeks on the SAFFA trial.

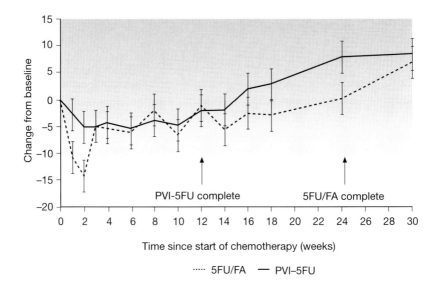

Figure 5.2 Quality of life throughout the chemotherapy period on the SAFFA trial.

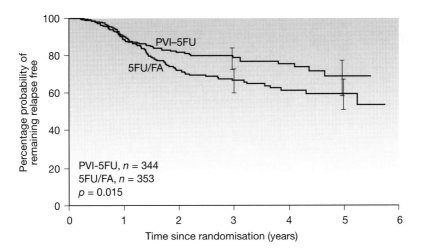

Figure 5.3 Relapse-free survival on the SAFFA trial.

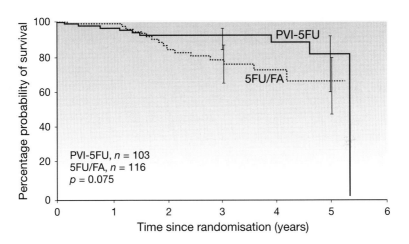

Figure 5.4 Overall survival in rectal cancers on the SAFFA trial.

Prognostic factors

There has for some time been considerable interest in developing new prognostic models that may better determine risk and/or predict chemosensitivity. This would permit a more rational approach to adjuvant treatment of colorectal cancer, in terms of both patient and drug selection. Areas of investigation include the prognostic significance of thymidylate synthase (TS) levels, DCC protein, microsatellite instability and the detection of micrometastases.

Table 5.5 Grade III–IV toxicity on the SAFFA trial

Toxicity	Bolus 5FU/FA (%)	PVI-5FU (%)	p
Diarrhoea	17	6	< 0.0001
Stomatitis	21	3	< 0.0001
Alopecia[a]	13	0.3	< 0.0001
Nausea/Vomiting	3	2	0.41
PPE	3	6	0.31
Anaemia	1.6	0.6	0.001
Neutropenia	55	0.6	< 0.0001

Saini *et al*. (2000).
FA, folinic acid; PPE, plantar–palmar erythema.
[a]Grade II.

TS levels and response to chemotherapy

Thymidylate synthase is the target enzyme of 5FU as well as newer agents such as Tomudex (raltitrexed). TS inhibition leads to the depletion of thymidine triphosphate (dTTP), thus interfering with DNA synthesis and repair. To date, studies investigating the significance of TS levels and response to chemotherapy have generally focused on response rates in metastatic colorectal tumours, and therefor some extrapolation is required to estimate its significance in the adjuvant setting. Leichman *et al*. (1997) performed polymerase chain reaction (PCR) on tumour specimens of 46 patients receiving infused 5FU for metastatic colorectal cancer. The ratio between TS and β-actin mRNA was available in 42 patients. TS levels greater than 4.1×10^3 predicted for resistance to 5FU. A TS level less than 3.5×10^3 was associated with a 52% response rate. Similar findings were described by Ford *et al*. (2000) after treatment with the specific TS inhibitor raltitrexed in patients with advanced colorectal cancer. Patients with a TS level greater than 4.1×10^3 in tumour tissue were significantly less likely to respond to treatment ($p = 0.02$). Interestingly levels greater than 6.6×10^3 in non-malignant tissue were associated with a significantly increased chance of grade II–IV gastrointestinal toxicity ($p = 0.007$).

The role of TS has been investigated in the adjuvant setting, however. Johnston *et al*. (1994) measured TS level in 294 patients with primary rectal cancer treated with surgery alone or surgery and adjuvant chemotherapy, in the context of the NSABP-R01 trial (Table 5.6). The 5-year disease-free survival rate in patients with low TS expression was 49%, compared with 27% in those with high TS expression ($p < 0.01$). The 5-year overall survival rate was 60% and 40% respectively ($p < 0.01$). In those with high TS expression, the 5-year overall survival rate after adjuvant chemotherapy or surgery alone was 54% and 31%, respectively ($p < 0.01$). No difference in survival was observed in patients with low TS expression. Thus, TS expression may be a potential marker for patients who benefit from adjuvant chemotherapy, particularly in those with otherwise favourable disease.

Table 5.6 TS expression and survival following adjuvant chemotherapy

TS intensity	n	Disease-free survival rate (%)	Overall survival rate (%)
Low	91	49	60
High	203	27	40
p		< 0.01	< 0.01

Johnston et al. (1994).

DCC protein

The allelic loss of chromosome 18q has been linked to prognosis in patients with stage II colorectal cancer (Jen et al. 1994). However, the exact gene deletion has not been identified. One possible candidate is the *DCC* gene (18q21.2) which is often deleted in colorectal cancer. Shibata et al. (1996) examined the prognostic significance of *DCC* gene deletion in resected colorectal cancer: 132 archival surgical specimens of stage II- and III-resected lesions were evaluated using immunohistochemical techniques. Half of the specimens were found to have detectable *DCC* gene. There was no significant correlation with sex, age, tumour location or TNM stage (Table 5.7). The 5-year overall survival rate was significantly superior in patients with DCC-positive lesions, in both stage II and III colorectal cancer (94.3% vs 61.6%, $p < 0.001$ and 59.3% vs 33.2%, $p = 0.03$ respectively). At completion of the study 64% of the cases with DCC-positive cancers were alive, compared with 33% of the DCC-negative cases ($p < 0.001$). In the multivariate analysis, only tumour stage and DCC status were found to be independent predictors of survival. The authors concluded that the absence of the *DCC* gene in stage III colorectal cancer predicts a poor outcome, but not to the same extent as in stage II cancers. They went on to suggest that evaluation of DCC status may identify the subgroup of Dukes' B tumours that would benefit most from adjuvant chemotherapy.

Table 5.7 DCC protein and prognosis in colorectal cancer

DCC protein	Dukes' B	Dukes' C
DCC positive (%)	94.3	59.3
DCC negative (%)	61.6	33.2
p	< 0.001	0.03

Shibata et al. (1996).

Microsatellite instability

Approximately 10–15% of colorectal carcinomas have widespread somatic alterations in the size of repetitive nucleotide sequences in their DNA, referred to as microsatellite instability (MSI). This phenomenon is caused by defective DNA mismatch repair, resulting from the inactivation of genes involved in the repair process. In those with hereditary non-polyposis colon cancer (HNPCC) syndrome, this is thought to result from a germline mutation in one of these genes, whereas in sporadic cases of colorectal cancer this is thought to be caused by transcriptional silencing of the *hMLH*-1 repair gene. MSI is more often detected in right-sided tumours, and in mucinous and poorly differentiated lesions, and is possibly linked to prognosis. Elsaleh *et al.* (2000) performed a retrospective analysis of archival material from patients with Dukes' C cancer to examine the influence of MSI on survival. Material from 646 consecutive patients (42% of whom received adjuvant chemotherapy) was examined using a PCR technique. As expected, MSI was found to be more common in right-sided rather than left-sided tumours (20% vs 1%), and occurred more frequently in women (10% vs 7%). The overall survival was found to be superior in those with MSI-positive specimens (58% vs 33%, $p = 0.043$). No difference in outcome was seen in patients not receiving chemotherapy (37% vs 32%, $p = 0.8$). However, the 5-year overall survival difference in patients who did receive adjuvant chemotherapy was highly significantly in favour of those with MSI-positive lesions (90% vs 32%, $p = 0.0007$) (Table 5.8). At the end of the study period, only 4% of patients with MSI-positive tumours died of their disease, compared with 40% who were MSI negative. Only sex and MSI status were found to be independent predictors of survival.

Table 5.8 Microsatellite instability (MSI) and 5-year overall survival rate

MSI status	All patients (n = 656)	No chemotherapy (n = 384)	Chemotherapy (n = 272)
Positive (%)	58	37	90
Negative (%)	33	32	35
p	0.043	0.8	0.0007

Elsaleh *et al.* (2000).

Detection of micrometastases

Immunohistochemistry studies have revealed that some histologically negative lymph nodes may in fact contain minute amounts of tumour, although the prognostic relevance of these findings is unknown. The reverse transcriptase PCR (rt-PCR) assay has been used to detect carcinoembryonic antigen (CEA) in tissues of patients with colorectal cancer. CEA is found in most colorectal cancers, but not in normal tissue. Liefers *et al.* (1998) employed the rt-PCR technique to elucidate whether the presence of CEA in histologically 'normal' lymph nodes of resected stage II cancers had any influence on survival. A total of 246 histologically normal lymph nodes from 26 consecutively resected stage II cancers were examined by this technique. Intact mRNA was extracted from 192 lymph nodes of the 26 patients. Micrometastases were detected in 36 (19%) of the nodes. Fourteen patients (54%) had at least one node positive. At the end of the study, 7 of the 14 'positive' patients had died of their disease (50%). Only 1 of the 12 'negative' patients had a cancer-related death (8%). The 5-year 'adjusted' survival rate (where only cancer-related deaths were considered) was 50% for those with micrometastatic disease, and 91% for those without ($p = 0.02$) (Table 5.9). The recurrence rate at 60 months was 8% in micrometastatic 'negative' disease, and 58% in cases with detectable CEA ($p = 0.02$). On multivariate analysis, only the presence of micrometastatic disease predicted independently for survival. The authors concluded that patients with Dukes' B tumours were a heterogeneous group with approximately half having an excellent prognosis, although the other half had a prognosis similar to patients with stage III disease.

Table 5.9 Micrometastases and survival in stage II colorectal cancer

Micrometastases	5-year adjusted overall survival rate (%)	5-year observed overall survival rate (%)
Yes ($n = 14$)	50	36
No ($n = 12$)	91	75
p	0.02	0.03

Liefers *et al.* (1998).

Novel agents in adjuvant chemotherapy for colorectal cancer

A number of novel agents have emerged with activity in colorectal cancer. These include raltitrexed (TS inhibitor), irinotecan (topoisomerase I inhibitor, CPT-11), oxaliplatin (a diaminocyclohexane platinum derivative) and oral fluoropyrimidines such as uracil–tegafur (UFT) and capecitabine. The majority of published trials to date have investigated their use in advanced colorectal cancer, but there are a number of ongoing studies in the adjuvant setting (Table 5.10).

Table 5.10 Current adjuvant trials for novel agents in colorectal cancer

Drug	Trial	Protocol
Irinotecan	PETACC-3	PVI–5FU ± irinotecan
	Intergroup	Bolus 5FU ± irinotecan
Oxaliplatin	MOSAIC	PVI–5FU ± oxaliplatin
	NSABP C-07	Bolus 5FU ± oxaliplatin
Oral 5FU	Roche	Capecitabine/FA vs 5FU/FA
	NSABP C-06	UFT/FA vs 5FU/FA

The PETACC-1 study was designed to compare bolus 5FU and raltitrexed (Ford & Cunningham 1999). It planned to recruit 2,800 patients with curatively resected colorectal cancer, but was closed prematurely as a result of an excess of drug-related fatalities in the raltitrexed arm.

Two ongoing studies are investigating the role of irinotecan in the adjuvant setting. PETACC-3 randomises between infused 5FU alone and 5FU with irinotecan.

The Intergroup study has a similar design, but 5FU is administered as a bolus rather than an infusion. Similarly the addition of oxaliplatin to 5FU is under investigation in two phase III studies, with 5FU administered according to an infusional regimen in one (the Mosaic study) and a bolus regimen in the other (the NSABP C-07 trial). Finally, both capecitabine and UFT (in combination with folinic acid) are being tested against a 5FU/folinic acid regimen in a Roche-funded study and the NSABP C-06 study respectively. The results of these trials are awaited with great anticipation.

Adjuvant radiotherapy

In most of these patients, radiotherapy is not an appropriate treatment modality. However, although outside the scope of this chapter, there is evidence that combined modality therapy is of benefit in rectal tumours. Studies are presently being conducted to evaluate the use of chemoradiation in patients with fixed or margin-positive colon tumours, especially in the caecum.

Adjuvant chemotherapy in elderly people

Data on adjuvant chemotherapy tolerability and benefits in older patients remain scarce, because this patient cohort is under-represented in clinical trials and results for older patients are seldom reported separately. In a recent publication, Popescu et al. (1999) analysed toxicity, response rates and survival in patients receiving chemotherapy in the adjuvant and palliative setting. Other than a higher rate of mucositis after adjuvant bolus 5FU, there was no significant increase in toxicity in those above the age of 70. After palliative chemotherapy, no significant difference was observed in the response rate, failure-free survival or 1-year survival in patients above or below the 70-year cutoff. These results suggest that elderly patients with good performance status tolerate chemotherapy and derive the same benefit as those below the age of 70.

Conclusions

The outlook for patients with resected colorectal cancer continues to improve, but several issues remain controversial. Despite the accepted value of adjuvant chemotherapy in Dukes' C colorectal cancer, its use in Dukes' B tumours remains unproven. However, a policy of individualised decision-making can be justified, such that it is frequently offered to fit patients, particularly those who have high-risk disease. 5-Fluorouracil has remained the backbone of adjuvant chemotherapy, but the optimal schedule has not been established. Publication of the SAFFA trial (Saint et al. 2000) has shown that the use of infused 5FU reduces toxicity while maintaining efficacy, and importantly confers a superior quality of life in comparison with bolus 5FU. If these results are confirmed, 3 months of infused 5FU may become the standard of care in these patients. New molecular prognostic markers should eventually allow a more rational and stratified approach to adjuvant chemotherapy, particularly with the advent of new agents that have activity in this disease. There is exciting potential for improvement in the treatment of patients with curatively resected colon cancer, and continuing preclinical and clinical research is required to reach this goal.

References

Anonymous (1995). Efficacy of adjuvant fluorouracil and folinic acid in colon cancer. International Multicentre Pooled Analysis of Colon Cancer Trials (IMPACT) investigators. *The Lancet* **345**, 939–944

Anonymous (1998). Toxicity of fluorouracil in patients with advanced colorectal cancer: effect of administration schedule and prognostic factors. Meta-Analysis Group In Cancer. *Journal of Clinical Oncology* **16**, 3537–3541

Anonymous (1999). Efficacy of adjuvant fluorouracil and folinic acid in B2 colon cancer. International Multicentre Pooled Analysis of B2 Colon Cancer Trials (IMPACT B2) Investigators. *Journal of Clinical Oncology* **17**, 1356–1363

Elsaleh H, Joseph D, Grieu F, Zeps N, Spry N, Iacopetta B (2000). Association of tumour site and sex with survival benefit from adjuvant chemotherapy in colorectal cancer. *The Lancet* **355**, 1745–1750

Ford HE & Cunningham D (1999). Safety of raltitrexed. *The Lancet* **354**, 1824–1825

Ford HE, Farrugia DC, Cunningham D *et al.* (2000). Thymidylate synthase mRNA expression may predict non-response in tumor and increased risk of toxicity in normal gastrointestinal mucosa following treatment with raltitrexed ('Tomudex'). *Proceedings of the American Society of Clinical Oncology* **19**, 243a

Jen J, Kim H, Piantadosi S *et al.* (1994). Allelic loss of chromosome 18q and prognosis in colorectal cancer. *New England Journal of Medicine* **331**, 213–221

Johnston PG, Fisher ER, Rockette HE *et al.* (1994). The role of thymidylate synthase expression in prognosis and outcome of adjuvant chemotherapy in patients with rectal cancer. *Journal of Clinical Oncology* **12**, 2640–2647

Leichman CG, Lenz HJ, Leichman L *et al.* (1997). Quantitation of intratumoral thymidylate synthase expression predicts for disseminated colorectal cancer response and resistance to protracted-infusion fluorouracil and weekly leucovorin. *Journal of Clinical Oncology* **15**, 3223–3229

Liefers GJ, Cleton-Jansen AM, van de Velde CJ *et al.* (1998). Micrometastases and survival in stage II colorectal cancer. *New England Journal of Medicine* **339**, 223–228

Mamounas E, Wieand S, Wolmark N *et al.* (1999). Comparative efficacy of adjuvant chemotherapy in patients with Dukes' B versus Dukes' C colon cancer: results from four National Surgical Adjuvant Breast and Bowel Project adjuvant studies (C-01, C-02, C-03, and C-04). *Journal of Clinical Oncology* **17**, 1349–1355

Moertel CG, Fleming TR, Macdonald JS *et al.* (1990). Levamisole and fluorouracil for adjuvant therapy of resected colon carcinoma. *New England Journal of Medicine* **322**, 352–358

Moertel CG, Fleming TR, Macdonald JS *et al.* (1995). Fluorouracil plus levamisole as effective adjuvant therapy after resection of stage III colon carcinoma: a final report. *Annals of Internal Medicine* **122**, 321–326

O'Connell MJ, Mailliard JA, Kahn MJ *et al.* (1997). Controlled trial of fluorouracil and low-dose leucovorin given for 6 months as postoperative adjuvant therapy for colon cancer. *Journal of Clinical Oncology* **15**, 246–250

O'Connell MJ, Laurie JA, Kahn M *et al.* (1998). Prospectively randomized trial of postoperative adjuvant chemotherapy in patients with high-risk colon cancer. *Journal of Clinical Oncology* 16: 295–300

Popescu RA, Norman A, Ross PJ, Parikh B, Cunningham D (1999). Adjuvant or palliative chemotherapy for colorectal cancer in patients 70 years or older. *Journal of Clinical Oncology* **17**, 2412–2418

Saini A, Cunningham D, Norman AR *et al.* (2000). Multicentre randomized trial of protracted venous infusion (PVI) 5-FU compared to 5-FU/folinic acid (5-FU/FA) as adjuvant therapy for colorectal cancer. *Proceedings of the American Society of Clinical Oncology* **19**, 242a

Shibata D, Reale MA, Lavin P *et al.* (1996). The DCC protein and prognosis in colorectal cancer. *New England Journal of Medicine* **335**, 1727–1732

Wolmark N, Fisher B, Rockette H *et al.* (1988). Postoperative adjuvant chemotherapy or BCG for colon cancer: results from NSABP protocol C-01. *Journal of the National Cancer Institute* **80**, 30–36

Wolmark N, Rockette H, Mamounas E *et al.* (1999). Clinical trial to assess the relative efficacy of fluorouracil and leucovorin, fluorouracil and levamisole, and fluorouracil, leucovorin, and levamisole in patients with Dukes' B and C carcinoma of the colon: results from National Surgical Adjuvant Breast and Bowel Project C-04. *Journal of Clinical Oncology* **17**, 3553–3559

Chapter 6

Scientific evidence and expert clinical opinion for the management of advanced colorectal cancer by combination chemotherapy

D Alan Anthoney and Matthew T Seymour

Introduction

For most of the last three decades, the development of chemotherapy for colorectal cancer has been a process of meticulous optimisation of single-agent therapy with 5-fluorouracil (5FU). Within this straightjacket, considerable progress has been made. Indeed, 5FU has turned out to be a more active and versatile drug than first imagined: it has a well-established evidence base for benefit in both the adjuvant and palliative setting, and when used well it lacks many of the distressing side effects of other cytotoxic drugs.

However, 5FU also has many limitations. For around a third of patients not even temporary stabilisation of disease is obtained, and over the past 10 years it has become clear that even the most active 5FU regimens, when subjected to the rigours of well-conducted, externally reviewed, multicentre, phase III trials, produce WHO objective partial or complete responses in fewer than 30% of patients.

In the early 1980s, Goldie and Coldman (1984) and others (Dexter & Leith 1986) developed models of tumour growth and response to chemotherapy incorporating the concepts of genetic and phenotypic instability, with the emergence of drug-resistant clones during treatment. Goldie and Coldman predicted that the results of chemotherapy would be improved by the use of concurrent or alternating drug schedules, provided that the individual agents were (1) independently active and (2) non-cross resistant. These ideas have underpinned the development of combination chemotherapy for most cancers, but could not be applied or tested in colorectal cancer because only one active agent, 5FU, was available.

At last, this situation is changing. Recent years have seen the arrival of two new drugs, oxaliplatin and irinotecan, each with the properties of independent activity and non-cross resistance, which are prerequisites for combination therapy in the Goldie–Coldman model. In addition, new evidence has emerged for an old drug, mitomycin, suggesting that it, too, may have a role in combination chemotherapy for colorectal cancer.

The rapid burgeoning of knowledge on the cellular and molecular basis of carcinogenesis and metastasis has held the promise of developing drugs targeted to specific components of the pathways involved. A wide range of agents is currently under development, with many reaching the stage of early clinical trials. Some of these agents have already displayed synergism with standard cytotoxic agents, suggesting that in the next few years there will be greater scope for combination chemotherapy in advanced colorectal cancer (ACC).

In this chapter, we review the current evidence for the non-cross-resistant activity of irinotecan, oxaliplatin and mitomycin C by looking at their use in patients with 5FU-resistant disease, and then we examine their role in first-line combination chemotherapy. We also briefly report on the results of trials of novel targeted therapies in combination with 5FU.

Drugs showing non-cross resistance with 5FU

Irinotecan

Irinotecan (CPT-11; Campto) is a semi-synthetic derivative of camptothecin. Its active metabolite, SN38, causes cytotoxicity through interaction with the endonuclease topoisomerase I (topo I). The normal function of topo I is to relieve torsion, which inevitably develops 'upstream' of the replication fork when DNA strands are separating during mitosis or transcription. When DNA is under torsional strain, topo I binds to it, makes a single strand break, and allows the nicked strand to rotate around the intact strand before re-ligating it (Figure 6.1). SN38 binds to the topo I–DNA 'cleavable complex', stabilising it and preventing re-ligation. This leads on to double-strand breaks when the replication fork collides with the cleavable complex.

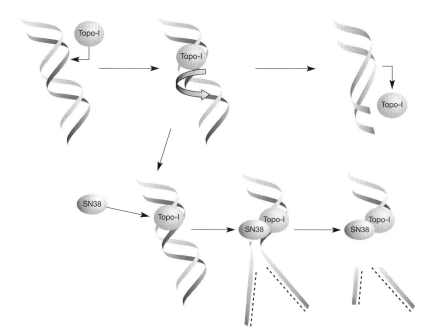

Figure 6.1 Mechanism of action of topoisomerase I (topo-I) and effect of the irinotecan metabolite SN38 (see text for explanation).

The pharmacology of irinotecan is illustrated in Figure 6.2. It is important, because several elements may lead to between-patient variability. Clearance of the active metabolite SN38 occurs through glucuronidation by UGT1A1, and biliary excretion of both SN38 and SN38 glucuronide, a process that involves transport systems such as P-glycoprotein and canalicular multi-organic anion transporter (cMOAT). Glucuronidation is reduced in patients with Gilbert's syndrome or Crigler–Najjar syndrome, and may be induced by drugs such as phenobarbital (phenobarbitone). Biliary excretion may be inhibited by various drugs including cyclosporin A, or by physical causes. SN38 in the small bowel may be responsible for the delayed diarrhoea which is one of the dose-limiting toxicities of irinotecan (Ratain 1998; Ratain *et al*. 1999).

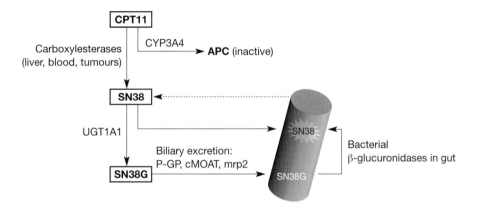

Figure 6.2 Pathways of activation and clearance of irinotecan (see text for explanation).

There is good clinical evidence that irinotecan, as a single agent, is an active drug in patients with 5FU-resistant disease. Randomised phase III trials of around 270 patients each were reported in 1998, both examining irinotecan at 300–350 mg/m^2 3-weekly for advanced disease progressing during or soon after 5FU therapy. In one trial the control arm was supportive care alone (Cunningham *et al*. 1998) and, in the other, an infusional 5FU regimen (Rougier *et al*. 1998). Both trials showed statistically significant survival advantages in favour of irinotecan with median improvements, respectively, of 2.7 months ($p = 0.0001$) and 2.3 months ($p = 0.035$). There is promising evidence that the significant toxicity of the 3-weekly schedule used in these phase III trials may be reduced by more frequent dose fractionation, or by pharmacokinetic modulation (Rothenberg *et al*. 1998; Ratain *et al*. 1999; Tsavaris *et al*. 1999). Irinotecan's non-cross resistance with 5FU is underlined by the fact that this second-line activity is obtained despite irinotecan being no more active than 5FU in non-pre-treated patients (Rougier *et al*. 1997; Saltz *et al*. 2000a).

Oxaliplatin

Oxaliplatin (L-OHP; Eloxatin) is a novel organoplatin that forms DNA adducts in a similar manner to cisplatin, but possesses a non-leaving group of diaminocyclohexane (DACH). The adducts formed are therefore distinct from other platins and the activity of the drug, both in preclinical models and clinically, is also distinct. One property of DACH–Pt adducts appears to be that, unlike cisplatin adducts, they are neither recognised by, nor dependent for cytotoxicity upon, the mismatch repair (MMR) protein complex (Figure 6.3) (Fink *et al.* 1996). This is of relevance since abnormalities of MMR are common in colorectal cancer and may confer resistance to other drugs such as 5FU (Barratt *et al.* 1998).

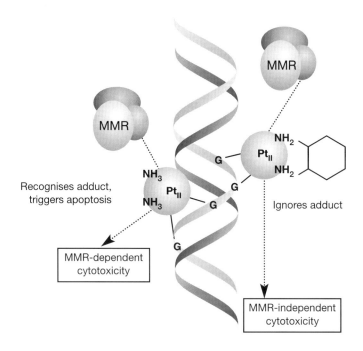

Figure 6.3 Contrasting effect of cisplatin–DNA adduct *(left)* and oxaliplatin–DNA adduct *(right)*. Unlike cisplatin, oxaliplatin adducts are not recognised by, or dependent upon, the mismatch repair (MMR) system.

For reasons that are not fully understood, oxaliplatin and 5FU interact synergistically in vitro. Therefore, clinical development of the drug has, from an early stage, concentrated on combinations with 5FU rather than single-agent therapy. Evidence for non-cross resistance of these combinations with single-agent 5FU/FA (folinic acid) comes from studies in which patients with documented disease progression on 5FU/FA alone were treated with oxaliplatin or oxaliplatin/5FU/FA.

Unlike irinotecan, there has been no phase III randomised trial to quantify the effect of second-line oxaliplatin on survival in this setting; however, phase II data are highly suggestive that its activity is at least as great. Large phase II second-line series include: (1) single agent oxaliplatin in 106 patients, with a reported objective response rate (RR) of 10% (Machover *et al.* 1996); (2) oxaliplatin added to fortnightly 5FU bolus plus infusion ('FOLFOX') in around 130 patients, with reported RRs of 20–40% and median survival of 10–16 months from starting second-line therapy (De Gramont *et al.* 1997b; Maindrault-Goebel *et al.* 2000); (3) oxaliplatin added to chronomodulated 5FU/FA in 67 patients, with RRs of 29–55% and median survival of 12–17 months (Levi *et al.* 1992; Garufi *et al.* 2000); (4) oxaliplatin added to the Mayo Clinic or AIO schedules in 172 patients, with an RR of 11% and median survival of 10.5 months (Van Cutsem *et al.* 1999). These data, although not randomised, are comparable with pooled phase II data for single-agent irinotecan in similar patient populations, where the RR was 13% of 363 (95% confidence interval or 95%CI 10–17%) and median survival was 9.5 months (Van Cutsem *et al.* 1997).

Mitomycin C

Mitomycin C has long been used in other gastrointestinal tract cancers, but its role in colorectal cancer is not clear. Three recent small studies have re-evaluated it in 5FU-resistant disease. Seitz *et al* (1998) reported a high RR and median survival of 10 months in 24 5FU-resistant patients treated with mitomycin plus the bimonthly bolus + infusion 5FU/FA, and our group obtained similarly good results with protracted venous infusion of 5FU + bolus mitomycin in 26 patients (Chester *et al.* 2000). However, a study of single agent mitomycin, given by 120-hour infusion, was less encouraging (Hartmann *et al.* 1998).

First-line combination therapy

After demonstrating independent activity against colorectal cancer and non-cross resistance with 5FU, the next logical step is to develop a combination chemotherapy schedule and compare it with single agent 5FU as first-line therapy. A general scheme for these investigations is shown in Figure 6.4. To date, two such trials are reported for irinotecan, two for oxaliplatin and one for mitomycin. The results of all five are summarised in Table 6.1.

Irinotecan/5FU combinations

The two trials involving irinotecan were presented at the 1999 American Society of Clinical Oncology (ASCO) meeting. Both were international, multicentre and large, one from the USA, Canada, Australia and New Zealand (Saltz *et al.* 2000a), and the other from Europe (Douillard *et al.* 2000).

In the American/Antipodean trial (Saltz *et al.* 2000a) 683 patients were randomised to bolus 5FU/FA alone, irinotecan alone or an irinotecan + bolus 5FU/FA combination.

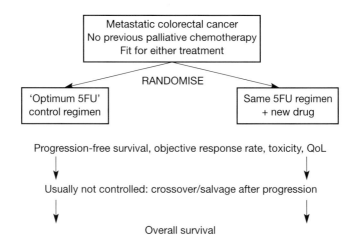

Figure 6.4 General schema for trials of first-line combination chemotherapy.

Table 6.1 Summarised results of first-line 5FU/LV ± irinotecan, oxaliplatin, mitomycin C, phase III randomised trials in advanced colorectal cancer

Reference	Treatment	n	RR (PR + CR) (%)	Median PFS (months)	Median OS (months)
Saltz et al. (2000)	Mayo 5-day 5FU/FA vs weekly 5FU/FA/ irinotecan vs weekly irinotecan	219 225 223	21 ($p = 0.001$) 39 18	4.3 ($p = 0.004$) 7.0 4.2	12.6 ($p = 0.04$) 14.8 12.0
Douillard et al. (2000)	5FU/FA (LV5FU2 or AIO) vs same 5FU/FA + irinotecan	187 198	23 ($p < 0.001$) 41	19 weeks ($p < 0.001$) 29 weeks	14.1 ($p = 0.031$) 17.4
De Gramont et al. (2000)	5FU/FA (LV5FU2) vs same 5FU/FA + oxaliplatin	210 210	22 ($p < 0.0001$) 50	26 weeks (NS) 36 weeks	14.7 ($p = 0.0003$) 16.2
Giacchetti et al. (2000)	5FU/FA (chrono) vs same 5FU/FA + oxaliplatin	100 100	16[a] ($p < 0.0001$) 53[a]	6.1 ($p < 0.05$) 8.7	19.9 (NS) 19.4
Ross et al. (1997)	Protracted infusion 5FU vs same 5FU + mitomycin	100 100	38 ($p = 0.024$) 54	23 weeks ($p = 0.033$) 34 weeks	($p = 0.033$)*

CR, complete response; OS, overall survival; PFS, progression-free survival; PR, partial response; RR, response rate.
*Not significant in the original paper. Updated analysis: Price et al. (1999).
[a]Includes confirmed as well as unconfirmed responses.

The design did not quite conform to the scheme in Figure 6.4, because the 5FU/FA schedule in the control arm (the Mayo clinic 5-day monthly schedule) differed from the weekly × 4 schedule used in the combination arm. Neither of these 5FU schedules can be regarded as 'optimum', the Mayo clinic 'control' regimen having proved to be substantially inferior to biweekly bolus and infusional FU/FA in a previous phase III trial (De Gramont *et al.* 1997a).

Irinotecan causes diarrhoea, neutropenia, myelosuppression and lethargy; one concern, therefore, was whether these overlapping toxicities would make the 5FU/irinotecan combination too toxic, although this was not the case. In fact, the toxicity of irinotecan plus 5FU was perhaps even antagonistic: the incidence of grade 3 or 4 diarrhoea was actually lower in the combination arm (23% of patients) than in the single-agent irinotecan arm (31%), despite using the same dose and schedule of irinotecan. Neutropenia was increased, but was still less than with the Mayo clinic 'control' regimen.

On the other hand, the anti-tumour effects were clearly not antagonistic: single-agent 5FU/FA and single-agent irinotecan gave almost identical progression-free survival (PFS) and RR, although results for the combination were significantly improved (see Table 6.1). The overall survival published in the final report of this trial was significantly better for the combination arm over the single-agent arms (Saltz *et al.* 2000a). However, this significant difference may in part be the result of multiple re-analyses of the trial.

The European trial (Douillard *et al.* 2000) involved 387 patients. These investigators wished to use an optimum 5FU/FA control regimen but, instead of agreeing a single schedule, they gave clinicians a choice of using either the French fortnightly bolus + infusion (LV5FU2) or the German weekly 24-hour infusion (AIO) regimen. With the latter, the dose of 5FU was reduced in the combination schedule.

The addition of irinotecan significantly increased toxicity compared with 5FU/FA alone, with neutropenia, fevers, diarrhoea, nausea and asthenia. However, the efficacy was also significantly increased, with improved time to progression and RR. In this trial, overall survival was also significantly increased despite the fact that 31% of control arm patients received irinotecan-containing salvage therapy, and patients in both arms received alternative drugs.

The two trials of 5FU/FA ± irinotecan have now been co-analysed. This predictably strengthens the statistical significance of the main study end-points, including survival (Saltz *et al.* 2000b).

Oxaliplatin/5FU combinations

Two trials of the design shown in Figure 6.4 have been reported to date. The larger was first reported at ASCO in 1998 (De Gramont *et al.* 2000) and updated at the 1999 meeting (Seymour *et al.* 1999): 420 patients were randomised to the 'LV5FU2' fortnightly regimen of bolus and infusional 5FU/FA with or without the addition of oxaliplatin. The addition of oxaliplatin increased toxicity, although this remained relatively mild. The characteristic toxicity of oxaliplatin is peripheral sensory neuropathy which, although very common, is mild and reversible in the large majority of cases. However, 18% of patients developed grade 3 neuropathy (involving pain or functional loss) and in a quarter of these (i.e. 4.5% patients) it was irreversible. It should be noted that the time to onset of significant neuropathy was > 4 months – much greater than the median time to response of 2.1 months. This ensured that patients who did not respond had been withdrawn from treatment before the onset of significant neurological toxicity. There was also significantly more grade 3 and 4 neutropenia with the addition of oxaliplatin (42% versus 5.5%), although only in 1% was this complicated by fever.

The efficacy of the combination was markedly improved, with highly significant increases in RR and PFS (see Table 6.1). Overall survival was not significantly affected, again perhaps explained by crossover and second-line treatment.

A previous, smaller study of similar design examined the addition of oxaliplatin to chronomodulated 5FU/FA (Giacchetti *et al.* 2000). Again, marked increases were seen in RR and PFS, although in this trial the control regimen produced a lower RR than in previous chronotherapy studies. Strangely, the control arm patients in this study enjoyed the longest median overall survival of all the trials reviewed, although the difference between the two arms was not statistically significant. A high proportion of the patients in both arms of this trial had subsequent hepatic surgery (26%). It is also worth noting that 57% of the control patients went on to receive oxaliplatin as second-line therapy, upon treatment failure, which raises the question of the optimum sequencing of therapies for this disease.

Mitomycin/5FU combination

Only one trial has asked the same question of mitomycin. It involved 200 patients randomised to continuous ambulatory 5FU infusion alone or with 6-weekly bolus mitomycin. The dose of mitomycin was reduced during the trial because of sporadic toxicity. This was a single-centre trial, and the RR of 34% to the control treatment was higher than expected. The combination arm had significantly better RR and failure-free survival. When first reported, survival was not affected, but a recent update now shows a small but significant survival advantage at 2 years (Price *et al.* 1999). In a subsequent randomised trial from the same group, 160 control arm patients received the same 5FU/mitomycin regimen with, once again, encouraging results in terms of failure-free survival (median 36 weeks) and overall survival (median 17.6 months), although RR was lower at 40% (Price *et al.* 1999).

The potential of mitomycin/5FU in the first-line treatment of ACC is reinforced by data from a large, multicentre, phase II study from Italy (Sobrero *et al.* 2001). The basis of this study is that fluoropyrimidines have different mechanisms of action depending on whether given by bolus or infusion, and therefore biochemical modulators should be specific for a given schedule. The regimen employed consists of alternating two biweekly cycles of sequential methotrexate (MTX) and bolus 5FU with 3 weeks of continuous infusional 5FU/LV and mitomycin C (MMC); 105 patients who had received no prior chemotherapy for advanced disease were treated with this regimen. The objective RR was 41% with a median duration of response of 8.1 months. Median failure-free and overall survival were 7.7 and 18.8 months respectively.

Although not a randomised trial, the authors suggest that their results and those above are important at a time when the focus is on new agent combinations. A comparison of the estimated costs of 6 months of treatment with the 5FU/MTX/MMC regimen and irinotecan/5FU shows the former to be significantly cheaper (Sobrero *et al.* 2001). This does not take into account costs associated with the treatment of drug-related toxicity which appears greater with the irinotecan/5FU combination. Although not directly comparable, objective RRs and PFS do not appear to differ greatly between combinations of 5FU and mitomycin C, irinotecan or oxaliplatin. It is therefore suggested that, in the euphoria of having novel agents to use in ACC, the search for alternative regimens of low cost and toxicity should not be discouraged.

New agents for advanced colorectal cancer: bullets for targeted therapy?

Despite the obvious excitement generated by the introduction of irinotecan and oxaliplatin into the range of therapeutic options for ACC, the search for additional active agents has been ongoing. Significant advances have been made in our understanding of the basic science of carcinogenesis and metastasis. In response to this, one of the aims of new drug development has been to target treatment specifically to tumour cells. Drugs such as capecitabine, which undergo activation within tumour cells, are one such form of targeted therapy. Over the past few years clinical trials on a number of other novel targeted therapies have been performed and results are beginning to appear.

Anti-angiogenic agents

Angiogenesis is a prerequisite for tumour development and metastasis. A pathway of particular interest in colorectal cancer is vascular endothelium growth factor (VEGF)-mediated angiogenesis. Evidence from preclinical and clinical studies has shown VEGF to be the predominant angiogenic factor in human colorectal cancer (Ellis *et al.* 2000). High levels of VEGF expression are associated with the development of metastases and a poor prognosis (Kumar *et al.* 1998), whereas expression of VEGF receptor (VEGFR) is greater in tumour than in normal vessel endothelium (Warren *et al.* 1995).

The use of monoclonal antibodies that bind and neutralise VEGF is one approach to anti-angiogenic therapy in colorectal cancer. Preclinical and early clinical studies have shown that a humanised recombinant monoclonal antibody to VEGF (rHuMab VEGF) can be administered with standard cytotoxic agents without increasing toxicity

(Gordon *et al.* 2001; Margolin *et al.* 2001). A randomised phase II study of rHuMab VEGF in combination with 5FU/LV was presented at ASCO (Bergsland *et al.* 2000): 104 patients with advanced colorectal cancer, either chemonaïve or more than 12 months after adjuvant treatment, were randomised to either 500 mg/m^2 5FU + 500 mg/m^2 leucovorin (LV) (weekly × 6 every 8 weeks) alone or in combination with low (5 mg/kg) or high (10 mg/kg) rHuMab VEGF (2 weekly until progression). Toxicity was primarily that expected with 5FU/LV and rHuMab VEGF was well tolerated. As seen in Table 6.2 the combination of 5FU and rHuMab VEGF would appear to increase the RR and time to progression in patients with untreated metastatic colorectal cancer over chemotherapy alone.

Table 6.2 Results of a randomised phase II trial of rhuMAb VEGF ± 5FU/LV in patients with advanced colorectal cancer

	5FU/LV (n = 36)	5FU/LV/l-d rhuMAb VEGF (n = 35)	5FU/LV/l-d rhuMAb VEGF (n = 33)
ORR (inv)[a]	7/35 (20%)	12/35 (34%)	12/32 (38%)
ORR (IRF)[b]	7/33 (21%)	13/31 (42%)	7/28 (25%)
TTP (inv)[a] (months)	5.4	6.8	7.3
TTP (inv + IRF[b]) (months)	5.2	9.2	7.2

[a]Investigator review.
[b]Independent review facility.
ORR, overall response rate; TTP, time to progression.

The VEGF receptors flt-1 and KDR are tyrosine kinases involved in signal transduction upon binding of VEGF. SU5416 is a receptor tyrosine kinase inhibitor that decreases VEGF-induced Flk-1 phosphorylation (Fong *et al.* 1999). Pre-clinical studies revealed that there was synergy between SU5416 and 5FU/LV (Rosen *et al.* 2000). A phase I/II study of SU5416 in combination with 5FU/LV given by the Mayo Clinic or Roswell Park regimen has shown this combination to be well tolerated, with toxicity predominantly that of the 5FU/LV (Rosen *et al.* 2000). Of 28 chemotherapy-naïve patients with metastatic colorectal cancer there were one complete response (CR), five partial responses (PR) and nine with stable disease. In an update presented at ASCO 2001 (Miller *et al.* 2001) the results of the study were compared with subsets of patients from the phase III clinical trial of 5FU/LV versus irinotecan/5FU/LV (Saltz *et al.* 2000a). The median time to progression for the SU5416 combination was comparable to those patients who received irinotecan/5FU/LV in the phase III trial. Phase III trials using 5FU/LV ± SU5416 and irinotecan/5FU/LV ± SU5416 are currently under way.

It has been shown that inhibition of VEGFR by SU5416 can lead to upregulation of other pro-angiogenic pathways, which could result in resistance to this agent.

The development of drugs that inhibit a number of pro-angiogenic pathways may be less prone to this problem and SU6668, which inhibits VEGF, fibroblast growth factor 2 (FGF2) and platelet-derived growth factor (PDGF), is currently in phase II trials.

Epidermal growth factor receptor inhibitors

Epidermal growth factor receptor (EGFR) is a transmembrane tyrosine kinase, which in association with one of its ligands, transforming growth factor α (TGFα), form part of an autocrine loop which stimulates expression of pro-angiogenic factors in cancer cells (Shawver 1999). In a large number of tumours EGFR status is altered, as a result of overexpression and/or mutation (Voldborg *et al.* 1997). This has been associated with an increased likelihood of metastasis, and hence poor prognosis, in colorectal cancer (Mayer *et al.* 1993).

Cetuximab (IMC-C225) is a monoclonal antibody specific for EGFR. Preliminary results of a phase II study of cetuximab in combination with irinotecan were presented at ASCO (Saltz *et al.* 2001). Tumours from patients with ACC, refractory to both 5FU and irinotecan, were screened for overexpression of EGFR by immunohistochemistry: 121 patients (72% of those screened) were treated with a 400 mg/m^2 loading dose of cetuximab followed by 250 mg/m^2 per week. This was in combination with the same dose and schedule of irinotecan that the patient had previously progressed on. Toxicity was mild to moderate (allergic and dermatological) and cetuximab did not appear to exacerbate irinotecan toxicity; 17% of patients showed a partial response (maintained for a median of 84 days), with a further 31% of patients showing minor responses or stable disease. Studies of cetuximab in combination with irinotecan and 5FU/LV as first-line treatment of ACC are ongoing.

A number of other agents that specifically block the tyrosine kinase activity of EGFR are currently in single-agent and combination clinical trials in colorectal cancer.

Cyclo-oxygenase 2

Cyclo-oxygenases (COX) are enzymes involved in prostaglandin biosynthesis. COX-2 is an inducible isoform not detected in most normal tissues, but upregulated in 85% of human colorectal carcinomas (Kargman *et al.* 1995). COX-2 has been shown to have a direct role in intestinal tumorigenesis (Oshima *et al.* 1996) and it has also been shown to be involved in neo-angiogenesis (Gately 2000), partly through upregulation of VEGF. Specific inhibitors of COX-2 have been developed that lack the gastrointestinal toxicity of previous non-steroidal anti-inflammatory drugs. It has been shown that the selective COX-2 inhibitors have anti-angiogenic effects and also induce cell cycle arrest and apoptosis in colorectal tumour cells (Elder *et al.* 1997; Tsujii *et al.* 1998).

To date the main thrust of clinical research with specific COX-2 inhibitors has been in chemoprevention or as an adjuvant after curative surgery. However, there are a number of specific phase II trials of COX-2 inhibitors in combination with cytotoxic chemotherapy currently accruing patients.

Conclusions

Until recently, we had only one useful drug for colorectal cancer: 5FU. Now, 5FU itself is being challenged by a range of pro-drugs and alternatives that may soon replace it (see Chapter 7), but more importantly we have at least two new agents with completely different mechanisms of action, which lack cross resistance and may feasibly be combined with 5FU. At long last we have entered the era of combination chemotherapy for colorectal cancer. The obvious next question is how to make best use of this new potential, both for patients with advanced disease and for those being treated with curative intent.

Where cure is a realistic goal, and the aim of chemotherapy is complete clonal eradication of cancer, the lesson from Goldie and Coldman, and from our experience in other cancers, is to use combination chemotherapy. Two-drug combinations as described in this chapter, but perhaps also three or even four-drug combinations, offer exciting potential to cure more patients with conventionally operable disease, and to bring more patients within the scope of curative surgery (Topham 2000). These schedules must be safe and deliverable without too much compromise to individual agent dose intensity, and the ongoing programmes of combination development in patients with advanced disease are the appropriate testing ground to establish new regimens and compare their efficacy. Three of the schedules established in the work reviewed here are already now under test in phase III adjuvant therapy trials.

When cure is not a goal, the aim of chemotherapy is to suppress the cancer burden below the threshold of symptoms and to keep it suppressed for as long as possible, i.e. to achieve the maximum possible extension of survival with good quality of life. It is possible that first-line combination chemotherapy will also be the best strategy to achieve this: the same principle of early suppression of all potentially sensitive clones may also be applied to non-curative therapy. However, this strategy carries a cost, both of finance and of toxicity, and will require testing.

If a patient has advanced disease and cure is not a goal, and if we plan to use more than one drug, should we give them together from the start, or use them sequentially? None of the trials reviewed sets out to answer that question; however, those testing first-line oxaliplatin or irinotecan combinations had 27–57% of control arm patients who crossed over to receive the test drug on progression. In one trial (Douillard *et al.* 2000), and a second (Saltz *et al.* 2000a), overall survival advantages have been seen, supporting the first-line combination approach, but not in the others. The trial with the highest rate of crossover also had the best survival for control arm patients (Giacchetti *et al.* 2000). The UK MRC is currently planning (running) a randomised trial which includes a randomisation to '5FU + new drug from the start' versus '5FU until disease progression, then add new drug' in an attempt to answer this question in a structured way.

Finally, a number of new agents, targeted to molecular pathways involved in carcinogenesis and metastasis in colorectal cancer, are showing promise in combination with standard chemotherapy. They raise the promise of even greater scope for the treatment of advanced colorectal cancer and the challenge of determining the best combination at the appropriate time for each individual patient.

References

Barratt PL, Seymour MT, Phillips RM *et al.* (1998). The role of hMLH1, a DNA mismatch repair gene, in response to anticancer agents currently used in the treatment of colorectal cancer, in an in vitro model. *Proceedings of the American Association of Cancer Research* **39** (Abstr)

Bergsland E, Hurwitz H, Fehrenbacher L *et al.* (2000). A randomised phase II trial comparing rhuMAb VEGF (recombinant humanized monoclonal antibody to vascular endothelial growth factor) plus 5 flurouracil/leucovorin (FU/LV) to FU/LV alone in patients with metastatic colorectal cancer. *Proceedings of the American Society of Clinical Oncology* **19** (Abstr)

Chester JD, Dent JT, Wilson G *et al.* (2000). Protracted infusional 5-fluorouracil with bolus mitomycin in 5FU-resistant colorectal cancer. *Annals of Oncology* **11**, 235–237

Cunningham D, Pyrhonen S, James RD *et al.* (1998). Randomised trial of irinotecan plus supportive care versus supportive care alone after fluorouracil failure for patients with metastatic colorectal cancer. *The Lancet* **352**, 1413–1418

De Gramont A, Bosset JF, Milan C *et al.* (1997a). Randomised trial comparing monthly low-dose leucovorin and fluorouracil bolus with bi-monthly high dose leucovorin and fluorouracil bolus plus continuous infusion for advanced colorectal cancer: a French Intergroup study. *Journal of Clinical Oncology* **15**, 808–815

De Gramont A, Vignoud J, Tournigand C *et al.* (1997b). Oxaliplatin with high-dose leucovorin and 5-fluorouracil 48-hour continuous infusion in pretreated metastatic colorectal cancer. *European Journal of Cancer* **33**, 214–219

De Gramont A, Figer A, Seymour M *et al.* (2000). Leucovorin and 5-fluorouracil with or without oxaliplatin as first line treatment in advanced colorectal cancer. *Journal of Clinical Oncology* **18**, 2938–2947

Dexter DL & Leith JT (1986). Tumour heterogeneity and drug resistance. *Journal of Clinical Oncology* **4**, 244

Douillard J, Cunningham D, Roth A *et al.* (2000). Irinotecan combined with flurouracil compared with flurouracil alone as first line treatment for metastatic colorectal cancer: a multicentre randomised trial. *The Lancet* **355**, 1041–1047

Elder DJE, Halton DE, Hague A *et al.* (1997). Induction of apoptotic cell death in human colorectal carcinoma cell lines by a cyclooxygenase-2 (COX-2) – selective nonsteroidal anti-inflammatory drug: independence from COX-2 protein expression. *Clinical Cancer Research* **3**, 1679–1683

Ellis LM, Takahashi Y, Liu W, Shaheen RM (2000). Vascular endothelial growth factor in human colon cancer: Biology and therapeutic implications. *Oncologist* **5**, 11–15

Fink D, Nebel S, Aebi S *et al.* (1996). The role of DNA mismatch repair in platinum drug resistance. *Cancer Research* **56**, 4881–4886

Fong TA, Shawver LK, Sun L *et al.* (1999). SU5416 is a potent and selective inhibitor of the vascular endothelial growth factor receptor (Flk-1/KDR) that inhibits tyrosine kinase catalysis, tumor vascularization, and growth of multiple tumor types. *Cancer Research* **59**, 99–106

Garufi C, Brienza S, Pugliese P *et al.* (2000). Overcoming resistance to chronomodulated 5-Fluorouracil and folinic acid by the addition of chronomodulated oxaliplatin in advanced colorectal cancer patients. *Anticancer Drugs* **11**, 495–501

Gately S (2000). The contribution of cyclooxygenase-2 to tumour angiogenesis. *Cancer and Metastasis Reviews* **19**, 19–27

Giacchetti S, Perpoint B, Zidani R *et al.* (2000). Phase III multicentre randomised trial of oxaliplatin added to chronomodulated flurouracil-leucovorin as first line treatment of metastatic colorectal cancer. *Journal of Clinical Oncology* **18**, 136–147

Goldie J & Coldman A (1984). The genetic origin of drug resistance in neoplasms: implications for systemic therapy. *Cancer Research* **44**, 3643–3653

Gordon MS, Margolin K, Talpaz M *et al.* (2001). Phase I safety and pharmacokinetic study of recombinant human anti-vascular endothelial growth factor in patients with advanced cancer. *Journal of Clinical Oncology* **19**, 843–850

Hartmann JT, Harstrick A, Daikeler T *et al.* (1998). Phase II study of continuous 120 h infusion of mitomycin C as salvage chemotherapy in patients with progressive or rapidly recurrent colorectal cancer. *Anti-Cancer Drugs* **9**, 427–431

Kargman SL, O'Neill GP, Vickers PJ *et al.* (1995) Expression of prostaglandin G/H synthase-1 and -2 protein in human colon cancer. *Cancer Research* **55**, 2556–2559

Kumar H, Heer K, Lee PW (1998). Preoperative serum vascular endothelial growth factor can predict stage in colorectal cancer. *Clinical Cancer Research* **14**, 1279–1285

Levi F, Misset JL, Brienza S *et al.* (1992). A chronopharmacologic phase II clinical trial with 5-fluorouracil, folinic acid, and oxaliplatin using an ambulatory multichannel programmable pump. High antitumor effectiveness against metastatic colorectal cancer. *Cancer* **69**, 893–900

Machover D, Diaz-Rubio E, De Gramont A *et al.* (1996). Two consecutive phase II studies of oxaliplatin for treatment of patients with advanced colorectal carcinoma who were resistant to previous treatment with fluoropyrimidines. *Annals of Oncology* **7**, 95–98

Maindrault-Goebel F, De Gramont A, Louvet C *et al.* (2000). Evaluation of oxaliplatin dose-intensity with the bimonthly 48hr leucovorin and 5-fluorouracil regimens (FOLFOX) in pretreated metastatic colorectal cancer. Oncology Multidisciplinary Research Group (GERCOR). *Annals of Oncology* **11**, 1477–1483

Margolin K, Gordon MS, Holmgren E *et al.* (2001). Phase 1b trial of i.v. rhuMAb to VEGF in combination with chemotherapy in patients with advanced cancer. *Journal of Clinical Oncology* **19**, 851–856

Mayer A, Takimoto M, Fritz E *et al.* (1993). The prognostic significance of proliferating cell nuclear antigen, epidermal growth factor receptor and mdr gene expression in colorectal cancer. *Cancer* **71**, 2454–2460

Miller LL, Elfring GL, Hannah AL *et al.* (2001). Efficacy results of a phase I/II study of SU5416 (S)/5-flurouracil (F)/Leucovorin(L) relative to results in random subsets of similar patients (Pts) from a phase III study of Irinotecan (C)/F/L or F/L alone in the therapy of previously untreated metastatic colorectal cancer (MCRC). *Proceedings of The American Society of Clinical Oncology* **20**, 571 (Abstr)

Oshima M, Dinchuk JE, Kargman SL *et al*. (1996). Suppression of intestinal polyposis in Apc delta716 knockout mice by inhibition of cyclooxygenase 2 (COX-2). *Cell* **87**, 803–809

Price T, Cunningham D, Hickish T *et al*. (1999). Phase III study of chronomodulated vs protracted venous infusional 5-fluorouracil both combined with mitomycin in first line therapy for advanced colorectal carcinoma. *Proceedings of the American Society of Clinical Oncology* **18**, 1008 (Abstr)

Ratain MJ (1998). New agents for colorectal cancer: topoisomerase-I inhibitors. In Perry MC, ed., *American Society of Clinical Oncology Educational Book*, 34th Annual Meeting, Vol 18. Alexandria, VA: American Society of Clinical Oncology, pp 311–315

Ratain MJ, Goh BC, Iyer L *et al*. (1999). A phase I study of irinotecan with pharmacokinetic modulation by cyclosporin A and phenobarbital. *Proceedings of the American Society of Clinical Oncology* **18**, 777 (Abstr)

Rosen PJ, Amado R, Hecht JR *et al*. (2000). A phase I/II study of SU5416 in combination with 5-FU/leucovorin in patients with metastatic colorectal cancer. *Proceedings of The American Society of Clinical Oncology* 19, 5D (Abstr)

Ross P, Norman A, Cunningham D *et al*. (1997). A prospective randomised trial of protracted venous infusion 5-fluorouracil with or without mitomycin C in advanced colorectal cancer. *Annals of Oncology* **8**, 995–1001

Rothenberg ML, Hainsworth JD, Rosen L *et al*. (1998). Phase II study of irinotecan 250 mg/m2 given every other week in previously treated colorectal cancer patients. *Proceedings of the American Society of Clinical Oncology* **17**, 1092 (Abstr)

Rougier P, Bugat R, Douillard JY *et al*. (1997). Phase II study of irinotecan in the treatment of advanced colorectal cancer in chemotherapy-naive patients and patients pre-treated with fluorouracil-based chemotherapy. *Journal of Clinical Oncology* **15**, 251–260

Rougier P, van Cutsem E, Bajetta E *et al*. (1998). Randomised trial of irinotecan versus fluorouracil by continuous infusion after fluorouracil failure in patients with metastatic colorectal cancer. *The Lancet* **352**, 1407–1412

Saltz LB, Cox JV, Blanke C *et al*. (2000a). Irinotecan plus flurouracil and leucovorin for metastatic colorectal cancer. *New England Journal of Medicine* **343**, 905–914

Saltz L, Douillard J, Pirotta N *et al*. (2000b). Combined analysis of two phase III randomised trials comparing irinotecan, flurouracil, leucovorin vs flurouracil alone as first-line therapy, of previously untreated metastatic colorectal cancer. *Proceedings of the American Society of Clinical Oncology* **19**, 938

Saltz L, Rubin M, Hochster H *et al*. (2001). Cetuximab (IMC-C225) plus Irinotecan (CPT-11) is active in CPT-11-refractory colorectal cancer (CRC) that expresses epidermal growth factor receptor. *Proceedings of the American Society of Clinical Oncology* **20**, 7 (Abstr)

Seitz J-F, Perrier H, Giovannini M *et al*. (1998). 5-Fluorouracil, high-dose folinic acid and mitomycin C combination chemotherapy in previously treated patients with advanced colorectal carcinoma. *Journal of Chemotherapy* **10**, 258–265

Seymour M, Tabah-Fisch I, Homerin M *et al*. (1999). Quality of life in advanced colorectal cancer: a comparison of QoL during bolus plus infusional 5FU/leucovorin with or without oxaliplatin. *Proceedings of the American Society of Clinical Oncology* **18**, 901

Shawver LK (1999). Tyrosine kinase inhibitors: from the emergence of targets to their clinical development. American Society of Clinical Oncology. *ASCO Annual Meeting Educational Book*, 35th Annual Meeting, vol 19. Alexandria, VA: American Society of Clinical Oncology, pp 29–47

Sobrero A, Guglielmi A, Cirillo M *et al*. (2001). 5-Fluorouracil modulated by leucovorin, methotrexate and mitomycin: highly effective, low-cost chemotherapy for advanced colorectal cancer. *British Journal of Cancer* **84**, 1023–1028

Topham CA (2000). Challenging the definition of 'best clinical practice': the impact of new and ongoing studies. In Cunningham D, Haller D, Miles A (eds). *The Effective Management of Colorectal Cancer.* London: Aesculapius Medical Press, pp 17–35

Tsavaris N, Ziras N, Kosmas C *et al*. (1999). Two different schedules of irinotecan administration in patients with advanced colorectal cancer relapsing after 5-fluorouracil leucovorin combination chemotherapy. Preliminary results of a randomised study. *Proceedings of the American Society of Clinical Oncology* **18**, 998 (Abstr)

Tsujii M, Kawano S, Tsuji S *et al*. (1998). Cyclooxygenase regulates angiogenesis induced by colon cancer cells. *Cell* **93**, 705–716

Van Cutsem E, Rougier P Droz JP *et al*. (1997). Clinical benefit of irinotecan in metastatic colorectal cancer resistant to 5FU. *Proceedings of the American Society of Clinical Oncology* **16**, 950 (Abstr)

Van Cutsem E, Bajetta E, Niederle N *et al*. (1998). A phase III multicentre randomized trial comparing CPT-11 to infusional 5FU regimen in patients with advanced colorectal cancer after 5FU failure. *Proceedings of the American Society of Clinical Oncology* **17**, 984

Van Cutsem E, Szanko J, Roth A *et al*. (1999). Evaluation of the addition of oxaliplatin (OXA) to the Mayo or German 5FU regimen in advanced refractory colorectal cancer (ARCRC). *Proceedings of the American Society of Clinical Oncology* **18**, 900

Voldborg BR, Damstrup L, Spang-Thomsen M *et al*. (1997). Epidermal growth factor receptor (EGFR) and EGFR mutations, function and possible role in clinical trials. *Annals of Oncology* **8**, 1197–1206

Warren RS, Yuan H, Matli MR, Gillet NA, Ferrara N (1995). Regulation by vascular endothelial growth factor in human colon cancer tumorigenesis in a mouse model of experimental liver metastases. *Journal of Clinical Investigation* **95**, 1789–1797

Chapter 7

Scientific evidence and expert clinical opinion for the optimal use of the oral fluoropyrimidines: combination therapy versus monotherapy

Paul Mainwaring

There is currently a series of changes in the management of advanced colorectal cancer that should improve the quality of life and the longevity of patients with this disease. Since its description over 40 years ago, 5-fluorouracil (5FU) has been the main chemotherapeutic agent around which systemic therapies for colorectal cancer have been based. Initial attempts to develop an oral 5FU preparation were hampered by its unpredictable oral bioavailability. Simultaneous inhibition of dihydropyrimidine dehydrogenase (DPD) has opened the possibility for safe, convenient and effective oral delivery of 5FU. Two other cytotoxic agents active against colorectal cancer have proved in the clinic to add benefit to the management of patients with advanced colorectal cancer. The next challenge is to combine the oral fluoropyrimidines with these novel chemotherapeutic drugs, irinotecan and oxaliplatin.

5-Fluorouracil

The half-life of 5FU is short at 10–20 minutes and the method of administration confers different benefit and toxicity profiles. The mechanism of action of 5FU is via incorporation in RNA as fluoro-uridine triphosphate (FUTP) and inhibition of thymidylate synthetase (TS) by fluoro-deoxyuridine monophosphate (FdUMP), often in conjunction with reduced folates for maximum efficacy to interfere with DNA synthesis. Importantly the ability of FdUMP to inhibit TS depends on its own concentration, as well as on the amount of functioning reduced folates. The rate of dissociation of the complex is inversely proportional to the concentration of reduced folate in equilibrium with the complex and, as intracellular reduced folate levels accumulate slowly when cells are continuously exposed to folinic acid (FA), so prolonged exposure may be needed to maintain its levels.

In advanced colorectal cancer, the aim is palliative except in the few patients with metastatic disease confined to the liver that is potentially resectable. Goals of therapy therefore focus on improving symptom control and minimising toxicity while at the same time trying to maximise the efficacy of systemic therapy. 5FU administered as a short (5-min) intravenous bolus affords response rates of approximately 10% in previously untreated metastatic colorectal cancer (Colorectal Cancer Meta-analysis Project 1992). These figures are improved by more than twofold with the addition of the biochemical modulator FA or by the delivery of 5FU in a variety of investigational delivery methods (Colorectal Cancer Meta-analysis Project 1992; Colorectal Cancer Group 2000). In advanced colorectal cancer, randomised studies have clearly shown that 5FU-based chemotherapy significantly prolongs survival. The results of the meta-analysis demonstrated that patients in the treatment group had a significantly reduced risk of death (hazard ratio 0.65 [95% confidence interval or 95%CI 0.56–0.76]). The absolute difference in survival was 16% at 6 months (79% vs 63%) and 12 months (50% vs 34%).

There are seven current commonly used 5FU delivery schedules, ranging from protracted continuous infusional 5FU delivery to bolus 5FU/FA delivery. Protracted infusional programmes of 5FU/FA delivery were developed in order to maximise the 5FU dose intensity. Investigators from the Mid-Atlantic Oncology Program compared daily bolus 5FU with a continuous infusion of 5FU delivered 24 hours a day for a protracted time (10 weeks or more) (Lokich et al. 1989). The response rate was 7% for the bolus arm and 30% for the infusional arm ($p < 0.001$). Toxicity was substantially different for the two arms, with leucopenia observed only on the bolus arm, including four sepsis-related deaths and hand–foot syndrome in the infusional arm, requiring treatment interruptions and dose reductions in a quarter of patients. In spite of the major difference in objective response rate, overall survival for the two groups was comparable.

A meta-analysis of six trials comprising over 1,200 patients examined the impact of infusional delivery schedules as a whole (Colorectal Cancer Meta-analysis Project 1998). Response rates of 22% for infusional schedules compared with 14% for bolus 5FU/FA ($p = 0.0002$), median duration of response of 7.1 months compared with 6.7 months, and overall survival of 12.1 months compared with 11.3 months (hazard ratio [HR] 0.88 [95%CI 0.78–0.99], $p = 0.04$), respectively, were reported. Short (24–48 hours) weekly/ biweekly infusional schedules of 5FU/FA delivery have reported very high response rates with reduced toxicity and consistently modestly improved survival benefits (Aranda et al. 1996, 1998; AIO 1997; de Gramont et al. 1998). Direct comparison of a 48-hour 5FU/FA infusion (LV5FU2) with the Northern Central Cancer Treatment Group (NCCTG)/Mayo regimen reported higher response rates, marginally higher median progression-free survival times and similar median survival times with reduced toxicity (de Gramont et al. 1997).

Oral fluoropyrimidines

The biochemical basis and rationale for the development of the oral fluoropyrimidines have been elegantly discussed at last year's meeting (Bissett et al. 2000). The identification of DPD inhibitors such as uracil and eniluracil has improved the predictability of the oral bioavailability of 5FU, enabling mimicry of the pharmacokinetics of protracted continuous intravenous 5FU administration.

For over 15 years, tegafur, a 5FU prodrug, has been administered for the treatment of gastrointestinal malignancies in Japan. In combination with uracil, UFT (uracil/tegafur) has demonstrated increased activity. Phase I and II trials in advanced colorectal cancer have established 300 mg/m^2 with 90 mg leucovorin three times daily as the therapeutic dose given for 28 days every 5 weeks. Two randomised trials were conducted comprising over 600 patients. Each study had a different control arm, one comparing to a 4-week Mayo regimen and the other versus a less dose-intensive 5-week Mayo regimen. Combining the results of the two studies demonstrated equivalent response rate and markedly reduced toxicity in comparison to the NCCTG/Mayo 5-day schedule (Table 7.1). Furthermore, in a crossover comparison 27 of 32 (84%) patients preferred oral UFT/leucovorin to the intravenous NCCTG/Mayo regimen (Borner *et al.* 2000). After having experienced both treatment modalities, patients taking the medication at home indicated less stomatitis and diarrhoea, and taking a pill rather than an injection as the most important reasons for their preference.

The second and currently most extensively employed of the oral fluoropyrimidines is capecitabine, a novel fluoropyrimidine carbamate that mimics continuous infusion 5FU. Capecitabine is metabolised to 5FU by a three-step enzymatic cascade and achieves tumour-selective generation of 5FU through exploitation of the higher concentrations of thymidine phosphorylase in tumour tissue compared with healthy tissue. Phase II trials have established a starting dose of 2,500 mg/m^2 per day given in two divided doses. It is given as a 3-week cycle, patients receiving 14 days of treatment followed by 7 days of rest. Two large randomised studies were carried out comprising a total of 1,207 patients, of which 603 were randomised to receive capecitabine. The two studies were identical in terms of study design, patient selection criteria, conduct and monitoring, and it was predefined that the data from both studies would be pooled.

Patients treated with capecitabine achieved a significantly superior response rate, which was demonstrated in all subpopulation analysis. In addition, capecitabine monotherapy demonstrated equivalent time to progression and overall survival. Capecitabine also demonstrated a superior safety profile with significantly less neutropenia, alopecia, diarrhoea and stomatitis compared to the Mayo regimen.

In summary, equally effective treatment may be safely delivered to patients with advanced colorectal cancer by substituting the NCCTG/Mayo bolus 5FU/FA regimen with either UFT/FA or capecitabine, as demonstrated in four large multicentre randomised trials (Table 7.1). Furthermore, considering the complexity and demands of bolus injections for 5 days every 4–5 weeks and the problems associated with insertion of central venous catheters such as infections, thrombosis as well as pneumothorax, delivery of therapy in the form of an oral fluoropyrimidine is much more convenient to patients and their carers.

Table 7.1 Randomised trials comparing oral fluoropyrimidines with NCCTG/Mayo 5FU/FA regimen

Study	Treatment	RR (%)	PFS (months)	OS (months)	p	G3–4 diarrhoea (%)	G3–4 mucositis (%)	G3–4 neutropenia (%)	G3–4 hand–foot (%)
Pazdur et al. (1999)	NCCTG 5FU/FA	15	3.8	13.4	NS	16	20	56	–
	UFT/LV	12	3.5	12.4		21	1[a]	1[a]	–
Carmichael et al. (1999)	NCCTG 5FU/FA	9	3.3	11.9	NS	11	16	31	–
	UFT/LV	11	3.4	12.2		18	2[a]	3[a]	–
Twelves et al. (1999)	NCCTG 5FU/FA	17.9	4.8	13.0	NS	10.0	13.4	19.7	0.3
	Capecitabine	26.6	5.3	13.7		10.0	Not stated	Not stated	16.2[a]
Cox et al. (1999)	NCCTG 5FU/FA	15.5	5.1	–	NS	13.9	16.3	25.9	0
	Capecitabine	23.2	4.4	–		15.1	Not stated	Not stated	17.7

[a]Statistically significant.
FA, folinic acid; 5FU, 5-fluorouracil; NCCTG, Northern Central Cancer Treatment Group; NS, not significant; OS, overall survival; PFS, progression-free survival; RR, relative risk; UFT, uracil/tegafur.

Oxaliplatin and irinotecan

One of two new compounds used for the treatment of advanced colorectal cancer is the novel platinum derivative oxaliplatin, which uses the addition of a lactone ring to enhance the inhibition of DNA repair and so increase cell kill. Oxaliplatin has modest activity as a single agent; however, there is strong synergy between its anticancer effect in combination with 5FU/FA, leading to high response rates when 5FU/FA is delivered as a short continuous infusion over 24–48 hours or by chronomodulated infusion (Graham *et al.* 2000). Two randomised trials have been reported comparing 5FU/FA with or without the addition of oxaliplatin. Giacchetti *et al.* (2000) reported improved response rates (including both confirmed and unconfirmed responses) and progression-free survival (8.7 vs 6.1 months), but no statistically significant difference in survival for the combined arm. In this trial 5FU/FA was delivered in the chronomodulated format (Table 7.2). Similarly, in the trial reported by de Gramont *et al.* (2000), combination chemotherapy was able to improve response rates significantly (50.7% vs 22.3%) and progression-free survival (median, 9.0 vs 6.2 months) but not overall survival (median, 16.2 vs 14.7 months). These two trials were powered for response and progression-free survival, respectively, and a significant proportion of patients received combination chemotherapy after progression on 5FU/FA – 57% and 37%, respectively.

Similarly, irinotecan has a novel mechanism of action by inhibiting the enzyme topoisomerase I. This enzyme is required for relaxing the twist in DNA before mitosis and has modest response activity when used as a single agent in advanced colorectal cancer (Bleiberg 1999). Two trials have demonstrated the superiority of irinotecan over 5FU and best supportive care alone in 5FU refractory disease (Rougier *et al.* 1998; Cunningham *et al.* 2000). More importantly, two randomised trials have now demonstrated a clinically significant survival advantage for the combination of irinotecan with 5FU/FA (bolus and continuous infusion) compared with the same 5FU/FA regimen. Douillard *et al.* (2000) used a combination of irinotecan and 5FU/FA delivered as a short 24- to 48-hour infusion over 1–2 days compared with 5FU/FA delivered in an identical manner, alone. There was a significant increase in response rates (49% vs 31%), time to progression (median 6.7 vs 4.4 months) and early separation of the survival curves (median 17.4 vs 14.1 months). A comparison of the Mayo/NCCTG regimen in combination with irinotecan to either treatment alone in patients with previously untreated advanced colorectal cancer has also been reported recently. The results of this trial also demonstrated a significant improvement in response rates (39% vs 21%), progression-free survival (median 7.0 vs 4.3 months) and overall survival (median 14.8 vs 12.6 months), albeit with a late separation of the survival curves. The majority of patients (56%) in the group given fluorouracil and leucovorin received an irinotecan-based regimen after the study.

Table 7.2 Randomised trials of combination chemotherapy compared with 5-fluorouracil/folinic acid

Study	n	Treatment	RR (%)	p	PFS (months)	p	OS (months)	p
Giacchetti et al. (1997)	100	Chronomodulated 5FU/FA	16	< 0.001	6.1	0.48	19.9	0.12
	100	Oxaliplatin + chronomodulated 5FU/FA	53		8.7		19.4	
De Gramont et al. (2000)	210	LV5FU2	22.3	0.0001	6.2	0.0003	14.7	
	210	Oxaliplatin + LV5FU2	50.7		9.0		16.2	
Douillard et al. (2000)	188	LV5FU2 or AIO	22	< 0.001	4.4	< 0.001	14.1	0.031
	199	Irinotecan + LV5FU2 or AIO	35		6.7 TTP		17.4	
Saltz et al. (2000)	226	NCCTG 5FU/FA	21	< 0.001	4.3	0.004	12.6	0.04
	231	Irinotecan + NCCTG 5FU/FA	39		7.0		14.8	
	226	Weekly irinotecan						

FA, folinic acid; 5FU, 5-fluorouracil; LV, leucovorin; NCCTG, Northern Central Cancer Treatment Group; NS, not significant; OS, overall survival; PFS, progression-free survival; RR, relative risk; TTP, time to progression; UFT, uracil/tegafur.

New combination therapies

Several reports have now looked at combining an oral fluoropyrimidine with the new colorectal cancer drugs.

In a phase I, dose-finding study 23 patients with advanced/metastatic solid tumours who had exhausted all standard therapeutic options received capecitabine/oxaliplatin combination therapy. In this study, the principal dose-limiting toxicity (DLT) was diarrhoea, which occurred in one of nine patients treated at the capecitabine 1,000 mg/m^2 dose level and two of six patients treated at the 1,250 mg/m^2 dose level. Partial responses were achieved in five of nine patients with advanced colorectal cancer, with a further three patients experiencing disease stabilisation. All patients had been pre-treated with 5FU-based regimens and four had received prior irinotecan. Therefore, capecitabine 1,000 mg/m^2 twice daily (days 1–14) combined with intravenous oxaliplatin 130 mg/m^2 (day 1), every 21 days, was identified as the recommended dose for further development (Diaz-Rubio *et al.* 2000; Evans *et al.* 2000).

Vanhoefer *et al.* (2000) conducted a phase I study of oral capecitabine twice daily on days 1–14, followed by a 7-day rest period, combined with weekly irinotecan (30-min infusion) for 6 weeks, repeated at day 50 in patients with measurable metastatic colorectal cancer as first-line chemotherapy. A total of 17 patients received 39 treatment cycles at three dose levels. The maximum tolerated dose (MTD) was reached at the third dose level: dose-limiting toxicities were grade 4 neutropenia (one patient), grade 3 diarrhoea (two patients) and grade 3 asthenia (one patient). Grade 3/4 neutropenia and grade 4 toxicities were observed only in the first treatment cycle and did not occur in subsequent cycles. There was only one further grade 3 adverse event (diarrhoea at dose level 1) and only one patient experienced hand–foot syndrome (grade 2, dose level 3). Four confirmed responses (one complete response and three partial responses) and six minor response/no change responses were observed in the first 17 patients. The study demonstrated that capecitabine/irinotecan combination therapy is feasible. The preliminary recommended dose for further clinical evaluation is capecitabine 1,250 mg/m^2 twice daily with irinotecan 70 mg/m^2. A phase II extension using the currently recommended dose level is ongoing to validate the regimen for phase III evaluation further (Vanhoefer *et al.* 2000).

Cassata *et al.* (2000) have examined the combination of capecitabine and irinotecan in patients with measurable advanced colorectal cancer. Irinotecan was administered at 300 mg/m^2 on day 1 every 3 weeks, or 150 mg/m^2 on days 1 and 8 every 3 weeks, followed by capecitabine 2,500 mg/m^2 per day, on day 2, for 14 days, followed by a 1-week rest period. Of the 19 patients, reported toxicities included were hand–foot syndrome (six patients, group 2 and one patient, group 3), nausea (one patient, group 3), vomiting (two patients, group 2), diarrhoea (seven patients, group 2) and neutropenia (two patients, group 2 and two patients, group 3). Partial responses have been observed in 13 of 17 response-evaluable patients (76%) with stable disease observed in two patients.

The combination of oxaliplatin and UFT/FA has also been examined. Seventy-one patients with previously untreated advanced colorectal cancer received oxaliplatin 85 mg/m^2 on days 1 and 14, leucovorin 250 mg/m^2 on day 1, followed by oral leucovorin 7.5 mg twice daily from days 2 to 14, with UFT 300–390 mg/m^2 per day twice daily on days 1–14, and with treatment repeated every 28 days. At the time of analysis, 34 patients were evaluable for response with 12 of 34 (35%) partial responses. Grade 3–4 diarrhoea was observed in 11 of 50 (21%) and grade 2–3 neurotoxicity was observed in 18 of 66 (27%) patients. As a result of the gastrointestinal toxicity, the recommended dose of UFT for this combination in 300 mg/m^2 (Dorta *et al.* 2000).

Seventeen patients with advanced colorectal cancer, who had failed at least one prior chemotherapy regimen, were enrolled in a phase I study using irinotecan administered on day 1, with oral UFT/FA administered on days 1–14, divided into three doses and with each cycle repeated every 3 weeks. The MTD was reached at level 3 (UFT 300 mg/m^2, FA 45 mg, irinotecan 300 mg/m^2), diarrhoea being the dose-limiting toxicity. Other observed toxicities included mild nausea/vomiting, asthenia, neutropenia, mucositis and alopecia. Of 13 patients evaluable for response, 4 had a partial response (31%) (Gravalos *et al.* 2000).

In another study designed to assess the MTD, toxicity profile and response rate of combination therapy UFT (250 mg/m^2 per day) and leucovorin (90 mg/day) were given on days 1–14, with escalating doses of irinotecan (200–300 mg/m^2) administered intravenously on day 1 of a 3-weekly cycle. Thirty-three patients with measurable, advanced colorectal cancer were enrolled. Initially, six patients were treated at each of the irinotecan dose levels of 200, 250 and 300 mg/m^2. One further patient was enrolled but not treated. Dose-limiting toxicities were observed in one patient at 250 mg/m^2 and three patients at 300 mg/m^2. These included diarrhoea and febrile neutropenia. Therefore irinotecan at 250 mg/m^2 became the recommended phase II dose and the cohort was expanded to 20 patients. Treatment at this dose was well tolerated with rates of grade 3–4 toxicity as follows: neutropenia 20%, diarrhoea 15%, fatigue 15% and nausea 10%. Response data for the first 16 patients reported one patient achieving a complete response (6.25%) and three achieving a partial response (18.75%) (Hill *et al.* 2000).

Eighteen patients who had previously received one line of chemotherapy for advanced colorectal cancer were entered into a study examining the combination of escalating doses of weekly irinotecan with a fixed dose of UFT (Escudero *et al.* 2000). Irinotecan was administered on days 1, 8 and 15 with UFT administered at 250 mg/m^2 per day for 21 days in two to three equally divided doses, every 4 weeks. The MTD was achieved when patients suffered from diarrhoea grade 4 (two events) and fatigue grade 3. Best response was recorded as stable disease in 12 of the 18 patients (66%). Median time to progression was 3.5 months. The recommended dose for phase II studies was weekly irinotecan at 110 mg/m^2 on days 1, 8 and 15 every 4 weeks with UFT 250 mg/m^2 on days 1–21.

With the improvements over bolus 5FU/FA delivery described above, investigators are beginning to report the results of combination chemotherapy using oxaliplatin or irinotecan with an oral fluoropyrimidine. Phase II trials are reporting consistently high response rates and survival comparable to those reported using combination chemotherapy based around short infusional 5FU/FA delivery. This approach could maximise therapeutic efficacy while minimising toxicity to provide the ideal therapeutic index for patients with advanced colorectal cancer.

References

AIO (1997). Biochemical modulation of weekly high-dose infusional (HD-CI) 5-FU in patients with advanced colorectal cancer. Results of a multicenter randomized AIO trial. *Proceedings of the Annual Meeting of the American Society of Clinical Oncology* **16**, A963

Aranda E *et al.* (1996). Outpatient weekly high-dose continuous-infusion 5-fluorouracil plus oral leucovorin in advanced colorectal cancer. A phase II trial. Spanish Cooperative Group for Gastrointestinal Tumor Therapy (TTD). *Annals of Oncology* **7**, 581–585

Aranda E *et al.* (1998). Randomized trial comparing monthly low-dose leucovorin and fluorouracil bolus with weekly high-dose 48-hour continuous-infusion fluorouracil for advanced colorectal cancer: a Spanish Cooperative Group for Gastrointestinal Tumor Therapy (TTD) study. *Annals of Oncology* **9**, 727–731

Bissett D *et al.* (2000). Optimal strategies for the use of oral fluoropyrimidines. In Cunningham D, Haller D, Miles D (eds) *The Effective Management of Colorectal Cancer*. London: Aesculapius Medical Press, pp 51–61

Bleiberg H (1999). CPT-11 in gastrointestinal cancer. *European Journal of Cancer* **35**, 19999

Borner M *et al.* (2000). A randomized crossover trial comparing oral UFT (uracil/tegafur) + leucovorin (LV) and intravenous fluorouracil (FU) + LV for patient preference and pharmacokinetics in advanced colorectal cancer. *Proceedings of the Annual Meeting of the American Society of Clinical Oncology* **19**, A741

Carmichael J *et al.* (1999). Randomized comparative study of Orzel® (oral uracil/tegafur (UFT™) plus leucovorin (LV)) versus parenteral 5-fluorouracil (5-FU) plus LV in patients with metastatic colorectal cancer. *Proceedings of the Annual Meeting of the American Society of Clinical Oncology* **19**, A1015

Cassata A *et al.* (2000). Phase I study of capecitabine in combination with a weekly schedule of irinotecan as first-line chemotherapy in metastatic colorectal cancer. *Annals of Oncology* **11**(suppl 4), 49

Colorectal Cancer Group (2000). Palliative chemotherapy for advanced colorectal cancer: systematic review and meta-analysis. *British Medical Journal* **321**, 531–535

Colorectal Cancer Meta-analysis Project (1992). Modulation of fluorouracil by leucovorin in patients with advanced colorectal cancer: evidence in terms of response rate. *Journal of Clinical Oncology* **10**, 896–903

Colorectal Cancer Meta-analysis Project (1998). Efficacy of intravenous continuous infusion of fluorouracil compared with bolus administration in advanced colorectal cancer. Meta-analysis Group In Cancer. *Journal of Clinical Oncology* **16**, 301–308

Cox JV *et al.* (1999). A phase III trial of Xeloda™ (capecitabine) in previously untreated advanced/metastatic colorectal cancer. *Proceedings of the Annual Meeting of the American Society of Clinical Oncology* **19**, A1016

Cunningham D, Falk S, Jackson DL (2000). Irinotecan and infusional 5-fluorouracil as first line treatment of metastatic colorectal cancer: improved survival and cost-effective compared with infusional 5-FU. *Proceedings of the Annual Meeting of the American Society of Clinical Oncology* **19**, A981

de Gramont A *et al.* (1997). Randomized trial comparing monthly low-dose leucovorin and fluorouracil bolus with bimonthly high-dose leucovorin and fluorouracil bolus plus continuous infusion for advanced colorectal cancer: a French intergroup study. *Journal of Clinical Oncology* **15**, 808–815

de Gramont A *et al.* (1998). A review of GERCOD trials of bimonthly leucovorin plus 5-fluorouracil 48-h continuous infusion in advanced colorectal cancer: evolution of a regimen. Groupe d'Etude et de Recherche sur les Cancers de l'Ovaire et Digestifs (GERCOD). *European Journal of Cancer* **34**, 619–626

de Gramont A *et al.* (2000). Leucovorin and fluorouracil with or without oxaliplatin as first-line treatment in advanced colorectal cancer. *Journal of Clinical Oncology* **18**, 2938–2947

Diaz-Rubio E *et al.* (2000). Phase I study of capecitabine in combination with oxaliplatin in patients with advanced or metastatic solid tumors. *Proceedings of the American Society of Clinical Oncology* **19**, A772

Dorta FJ *et al.* (2000). Phase II clinical trial with the combination of oxaliplatin-UFT-l, -leucovorin (OXA-UFT-l, LV) for the first line treatment of advanced colorectal cancer (ACC). Preliminary results (Oncopaz Cooperative Group – Spain). *Annals of Oncology* **11**(suppl 4), 50

Douillard J-Y *et al.* (2000). Irinotecan combined with fluorouracil compared with fluorouracil alone as first-line treatment for metastatic colorectal cancer: a multicentre randomised trial. *The Lancet* **355**, 1041–1047

Escudero P *et al.* (2000). Phase I–II trial of irinotecan (CPT-11) over a short IV weekly infusion combined with a fixed dose of UFT in second line advanced colorectal carcinoma (ACRC). *Proceedings of the Annual Meeting of the American Society of Clinical Oncology* **19**, A1136

Evans J *et al.* (2000). Safety profile and preliminary efficacy of capecitabine (Xeloda®) in combination with oxaliplatin in patients with advanced or metastatic solid tumours: Results from a phase I study. *Annals of Oncology* **11**(suppl 4), 51

Giacchetti S *et al.* (1997). Phase III trial of 5-fluorouracil (5-FU), folinic acid (FA), with or without oxaliplatin (OXA) in previously untreated patients (pts) with metastatic colorectal cancer (MCC) (Meeting abstract). *Proceedings of the Annual Meeting of the American Society of Clinical Oncology* **16**

Giacchetti S *et al.* (2000). Phase III multicenter randomized trial of oxaliplatin added to chronomodulated fluorouracil-leucovorin as first-line treatment of metastatic colorectal cancer. *Journal of Clinical Oncology* **18**, 136–147

Graham MA *et al.* (2000). Clinical pharmacokinetics of oxaliplatin: a critical review. *Clinical Cancer Research* **6**, 1205–1218

Gravalos C *et al.* (2000). Phase I trial of escalating doses of irinotecan (CPT-11) in combination with UFT/folinic acid (FA) in patients with advanced colorectal cancer (CRC). *Annals of Oncology* **11**(suppl 4), 46

Hill M *et al.* (2000). A phase i/ii study of oral uracil/tegafur (UFT) plus leucovorin (LV) combined with irinotecan (CPT-11) in patients with advanced or metastatic colorectal cancer (CRC). *Proceedings of the Annual Meeting of the American Society of Clinical Oncology* **20**, A1004

Lokich JJ *et al.* (1989). A prospective randomized comparison of continuous infusion fluorouracil with a conventional bolus schedule in metastatic colorectal carcinoma: a Mid-Atlantic Oncology Program Study. *Journal of Clinical Oncology* **7**, 425–432

Mani S *et al.* (2000). Multicenter phase II study to evaluate a 28-day regimen of oral fluorouracil plus eniluracil in the treatment of patients with previously untreated metastatic colorectal Cancer. *Journal of Clinical Oncology* **15**, 2894–3001

Pazdur R *et al.* (1999). Multicenter phase III study of 5-fluorouracil (5-FU) or UFTTM in combination with leucovorin (LV) in patients with metastatic colorectal cancer. *Proceedings of the Annual Meeting of the American Society of Clinical Oncology* **19**, A1009

Rougier P *et al.* (1998). Randomised trial of irinotecan versus fluorouracil by continuous infusion after fluorouracil failure in patients with metastatic colorectal cancer. *The Lancet* **352**, 1407–1412

Saltz LB *et al.* (2000). Irinotecan plus fluorouracil and leucovorin for metastatic colorectal cancer. *New England Journal of Medicine* **343**

Twelves C *et al.* (1999). A phase III trial (S014796) of Xeloda™ (capecitabine) in previously untreated advanced/metastatic colorectal cancer. *Proceedings of the Annual Meeting of the American Society of Clinical Oncology* **19**, A1010

Vanhoefer U *et al.* (2000) Phase I study of capecitabine in combination with a weekly schedule of irinotecan (CPT-11) as first-line chemotherapy in metastatic colorectal cancer. *Proceedings of the Annual Meeting of the American Society of Clinical Oncology* **19**, A1059

Chapter 8

Novel strategies for the treatment of colorectal cancer

Daniel Hochhauser

Introduction

There have been recent significant advances in the treatment of advanced colorectal cancer (CRC). The topoisomerase I (topo I) poison irinotecan (CPT-11) demonstrates activity in advanced disease and has been shown to prolong survival as both first- and second-line treatment settings (Cunningham *et al.* 1998; Douillard *et al.* 2000). In addition oxaliplatin shows significant activity in both chemotherapy-naïve and previously treated patients. These agents are also currently under evaluation in both the neoadjuvant and adjuvant settings. Despite these promising results, there are important problems with conventional chemotherapeutic agents. Both intrinsic and acquired resistance to these agents has been demonstrated through a great variety of mechanisms. In addition, the lack of specificity of conventional DNA-interacting agents results in significant systemic toxicities.

Over the past decade, there has been a dramatic increase in understanding of the molecular factors resulting in the development and progression of colon cancer. This has led to the identification of new targets for therapy which can be investigated rationally. This article summarises several novel and promising approaches to the treatment of advanced colorectal cancer (CRC) but is not intended to be exhaustive.

Modulation of chemosensitivity

It would clearly be of benefit to understand the reasons why particular agents such as CPT-11, oxaliplatin and fluorouracil have activity in CRC. There has been extensive work to define the factors that may predict sensitivity to these agents. This has been of most benefit in the case of fluorouracil where numerous studies have demonstrated a correlation between the level of thymidylate synthase (TS) expression and response to treatment (Johnston *et al.* 1995; Paradiso *et al.* 2000). Tumours with high levels of TS have a low probability of response to fluorouracil and there may be an increasing role for pre-treatment quantitation of TS levels. Defects in the process of mismatch repair may play a role in determining sensitivity to oxaliplatin (see below). The factors that determine sensitivity to topo I inhibitors are not well understood. Although increased levels of topo I in vitro are associated with increased sensitivity to CPT-11, this has not been confirmed in clinical studies. This is probably because there are multiple pathways by which these agents induce apoptosis and it may be simplistic to measure a single variable such as topo I levels. Furthermore, consistent and accurate measurement of topo I levels is difficult. However, it has been shown that levels of topo I decline following drug treatment as a result of activation of the ubiquitin/ proteasome pathway which regulates the degradation of intracellular proteins. This decline may be abrogated by specific proteasome inhibitors. The 26-S proteasome inhibitor MG132 was shown to inhibit CPT-11-induced downregulation of topo I in CRC cells and selectively sensitised cells to CPT-11-induced cytotoxicity and apoptosis (Desai *et al.* 2001). These agents may act in part by maintaining topo I levels and consequently increasing the number of drug-induced DNA strand breaks.

It is unlikely therefore that examination of the expression profiles of single genes will allow accurate prognostic predictions to be made. The increasing sophistication of DNA microarrays allows the identification of gene clusters that indicate prognosis as well as the responses to specific agents. Such an approach has already been of value in cell lines and clinically in analysing expression of genes after drug treatment (Kudoh *et al.* 2000). In CRC cells, clusters of gene expression have been uncovered by microarrays, suggesting the presence of organised patterns of gene expression, which could be used to classify tumours (Alon *et al.* 1999). Such studies will complement conventional pathological techniques in the future (Aparicio *et al.* 2000) and will allow more accurate prediction of chemosensitivity than measurement of the expression levels of individual genes.

Drug resistance and colorectal cancer

There has been extensive study of the significance of P-glycoprotein (PGP) expression in human cancers. PGP acts as an efflux pump with substrates including vinca alkaloids and doxorubicin. Alkylating agents do not induce expression of the multidrug-resistant (MDR) phenotype. Increased expression of PGP may indicate a poorer prognosis independent of treatment, as well as predicting resistance to chemotherapy (Kaye 1998). High levels of PGP expression occur in CRC and this may contribute partially to the intrinsic resistance to agents such as taxanes and anthracyclines. There is evidence of the efficacy of MDR inhibitors such as the cyclosporin analogue PSC-833 in the treatment of acute myeloid leukaemias (Advani *et al.* 1999), but PGP-reversal agents have not been fully evaluated in CRC. It will be important to investigate whether PGP-related proteins, such as the multidrug resistance protein (MRP), are factors in the intrinsic drug resistance of CRC before testing novel inhibitors. Such information will be obtained by microarray datasets of CRC cells before and after drug treatment.

There is a clear relationship between resistance to platinum agents and deficiencies in mismatch repair. Deficiency in mismatch repair occurs frequently in CRC and germline loss is associated with the hereditary non-polyposis colon cancer (*HNPCC*) phenotype. Loss of mismatch repair correlates with resistance to *cis*-platinum in vitro. The reasons for this are unclear but may be the result of the lethality of replicative bypass of platinum crosslinks in mismatch repair-proficient cells (Vaisman *et al.* 1998). Interestingly, there is no involvement of the mismatch repair pathway in processing of lesions induced by oxaliplatin (Fink *et al.* 1996). Genes for mismatch repair proteins such as hMLH1 are frequently downregulated by promoter methylation in CRC cells and the use of inhibitors such as the demethylating agent 2′-deoxy-5-azacytidine (DAC) can induce expression of mismatch repair proteins (Strathdee *et al.* 1999). There is consequently sensitisation of cells to platinum compounds.

Novel agents interacting with DNA

Many of the novel strategies in CRC involve molecular targeting of genes specifically expressed in human cancers. The recent results with CPT-11 and oxaliplatin indicate that there is a continuing important role for agents that interact with DNA. Several DNA-interacting agents are currently in advanced preclinical and clinical development. Ecteinascidin (ET-743) is a derivative of a murine tunicate which interacts with the minor groove of DNA (Zewail-Foote & Hurley 1999). ET-743 selectively alkylates guanine in the minor groove of duplex DNA and bends the DNA towards the major groove. The action of this agent is independent of topo I and was shown to have activity against a colon cancer cell line; there is clinical activity in soft tissue sarcomas (Delaloge *et al.* 2001) and ongoing clinical evaluation of ET-743 in CRC.

Alkylating agents have limited sequence specificity and increasing specificity for specific DNA sequences may enhance cytotoxicity. Furthermore, there is less efficient repair of damage by drugs that interact within the minor groove of DNA. These factors allow the development of more potent DNA-interacting drugs. A novel sequence-selective pyrrolobenzodiazepine (PBD) dimer, SJG-136, has been developed and is a highly efficient, minor groove interstrand, DNA-crosslinking agent that is 440-fold more potent than melphalan (Gregson *et al.* 2001). Although SJG-136 is still in preclinical evaluation, there is clearly major scope for developing more potent DNA-interacting agents.

Alkylating agents have been shown to have minimal activity in CRC and there is no evidence that dose intensification is of value. However, the strategy of antibody-directed enzyme pro-drug therapy (ADEPT) allows a significantly increased drug concentration to be achieved at the site of the cancer. This approach depends on the synthesis of antibodies to tumour-specific antigens such as carcinoembryonic antigen (CEA) which are linked either chemically or by recombinant techniques to an enzyme. Subsequent to injection of the antibody–enzyme complex, an intrinsically inactive pro-drug is administered and this is enzymatically converted to active drug at the site of the tumour. Therefore, high concentrations of drug are obtained at the site of the tumour with the advantage of bystander activity against cells not expressing the antigen. Systemic toxicity is reduced by both dilutional effects and the short half-life of the activated pro-drug. A clinical study of ADEPT has been carried out in CRC using a carboxypeptidase enzyme which activates a nitrogen mustard pro-drug to active drug (Napier *et al*. 2000). This and subsequent trials have shown the feasibility of this approach, as well as providing preliminary evidence of efficacy in terms of both demonstration of interstrand crosslinks within cancer cells and tumour response (Webley *et al*. 2001).

There are several strategies under development of small molecules that target DNA and mRNA. Antisense oligonucleotides are unmodified or chemically modified single-stranded DNA molecules, which hybridise to specific mRNAs of individual genes and inhibit mRNA function and gene expression. This approach has already been shown to be clinically feasible in the reduction of tumour *bcl*2 mRNA levels in non-Hodgkin's lymphoma (Waters *et al*. 2000). Several preclinical studies demonstrate the potential of this strategy in the context of molecular targeting of CRC, including antisense oligonucleotides to *bcl*2 and the RI-α regulatory subunit of protein kinase A, which increase chemosensitivity of cell lines. A phase II clinical trial of an antisense oligonucleotide to the translation initiation site of H-*ras* mRNA is in progress for patients with advanced CRC.

There is increasing interest in direct targeting of either the promoters or coding regions of genes dysregulated in cancer by development of sequence-specific DNA-interacting agents. This has involved the development of a new and effective class of DNA sequence-recognition molecules known as polyamides. These molecules can be designed by combinations of imidazole and pyrrole moieties to bind defined purine–pyrimidine sequences (Dervan & Burli 1999). This, for example, allows the binding site for the *ets* transcription factor promoter within the Her-2-*neu* promoter to be specifically targeted in vitro (Chiang *et al*. 2000). The other approach involves refinement of the PBD moiety to allow covalent binding to specific sequences within the minor groove of DNA. Several such agents, such as the highly selective DNA-interactive molecule CC-1065, have been produced; these molecules show cytotoxic activity at nanomolar concentrations. Critical issues include the cellular permeability of these molecules and the necessity of increasing the number of nucleotides targeted to improve specificity. These drugs will potentially modulate gene expression within tumours. Strategies for nucleic acid targeting are well summarised in Thurston (1999).

Molecular targeting of colorectal cancer
p53 and *ras*

There has been extensive progress in recent years in defining the molecular pathways occurring in the progression of CRC. It has become clear that mutation or deletion of several critical genes including *p53*, *ras* and *APC* are essential for the development of CRC. These pathways are described in Kinzler and Vogelstein (1996).

The p53 protein is mutated or deleted in up to 70% of CRC. Introduction of wild-type *p53* into cancer cells results in activation of apoptosis and sensitisation to chemotherapy. Several gene therapy protocols for colon cancer are under development, but problems remains in vector design and gene delivery (Chung-Faye *et al.* 2000). A phase I study of *p53* gene therapy using recombinant adenovirus in advanced CRC has demonstrated detectable transgene expression. Another strategy that exploits the absence of wild-type *p53* is administration of a mutated adenovirus which replicates and has a cytolytic effect only in the presence of mutant *p53*. Onyx-015 – an E1B 55-kilodalton (kDa), gene-deleted adenovirus – has been tested in 200 cancer patients in over 10 clinical trials (Kirn 2001). Clinical studies in combination with chemotherapy in head and neck cancer (Khuri *et al.* 2000) have confirmed that replicating adenovirus can be detected and there is evidence of clinical activity. In view of the high incidence of mutated *p53* in CRC, this will clearly be an optimal target.

Another gene product of considerable therapeutic interest is the *ras* oncogene (Adjei 2001). Mutation of the K-*ras* oncogene is found in over 40% of cases of CRC. There is essential post-translational modification of *ras* known as farnesylation, which is required for the oncogenic effects of *ras*. Inhibitors of farnesyltransferase (FTI) have been shown in vitro to reverse the effects of *ras*-induced cellular proliferation and have demonstrated clinical activity in leukaemias and solid tumours, although these agents may also affect the processing of other proteins including nuclear lamins. Current phase III studies of FTI are under way in CRC. *Ras*-induced cellular proliferation requires downstream activation of several components including the c-*Raf* kinase that has been inhibited by both antisense oligonucleotides and small molecules in vitro, and is currently in clinical phase II studies. Furthermore, inhibitors of the downstream MAPK kinase (MAPKK or MEK1) significantly inhibit CRC cell-line proliferation. These studies confirm that increased understanding of the molecular pathways involved in cancer cell proliferation can guide the development of novel anticancer agents.

Another approach to the inhibition of signal transduction pathways in cancer has been in the synthesis of the geldanamycins. These drugs target the heat shock protein Hsp-90, a chaperone protein required for protein stability of several gene products, including *ras* and *raf*. The agent 17-allylamino-17-demethoxygeldanamycin (17AAG) can reduce levels of N-*ras* and Ki-*ras* and induce apoptosis in CRC cells; it is now entering clinical trials (Hostein *et al.* 2001).

Cell cycle genes

In common with other cancers there is deregulation of cell cycle control in CRC (Nevins 2001). Several alterations occur, including mutation of the retinoblastoma protein, overexpression of cyclin D1 and mutation of the cyclin-dependent kinase inhibitor p16. In each of these cases, the normal controls on cell cycle progression are deficient. It can be shown in vitro that inhibition of components of the cell cycle such as the cyclin-dependent kinases (CDKs) results in apoptosis or may sensitise cancer cells to chemotherapy. The CDKs regulate progression through the cell cycle at the transition from G1 to S phases, and progression through S. There are several ATP site-directed inhibitors, including flavopiridol, *N*-substituted adenine derivatives, the natural product butyrolactone, staurosporin derivatives, and, more recently, the synthetic paullones (Senderowicz 2000). The most widely studied is the CDK inhibitor flavopiridol which induces cell cycle arrest after binding to multiple CDKs. There is synergy between paclitaxel and flavopiridol, in which the accelerated exit of cells from mitosis sensitises to the CDK inhibitor. Several studies are investigating the potential for combinations of flavopiridol with a variety of drugs including CPT-11.

Cyclo-oxygenase inhibition

There have been several epidemiological studies demonstrating a reduction in the incidence in CRC in patients using non-steroidal anti-inflammatory drugs (NSAIDs). These agents work through the inhibition of cyclo-oxygenases (COX) 1 and 2. COX-2 has been demonstrated to be upregulated in 40% of colorectal adenomas and 80% of cases of CRC. A novel class of specific COX-2 inhibitors has been developed that induce cell cycle arrest and apoptosis in CRC cells, as well as having anti-angiogenic properties (Fitzgerald & Patron 2001). Celecoxib, a specific COX-2 inhibitor, has been shown in a randomised study to reduce the incidence of colorectal polyps in patients with familial adenomatous polyposis (Steinbach *et al.* 2000). These agents are currently undergoing clinical trials in both chemoprevention and therapeutic contexts for CRC.

Growth factor receptors

As with other solid tumours such as breast cancer, growth factor membrane receptors of the transmembrane kinase family may be upregulated in CRC. These include the epidermal growth factor receptor (EGFR) which is upregulated in around 70% of cases of CRC. There have been approaches including antibodies to EGFR, small molecules inhibiting dimerisation of the intracellular domain and antisense oligonucleotides (Mendelsohn & Baselga 2000). Both inhibition of proliferation and induction of apoptosis have been demonstrated preclinically in a variety of cellular models. There is notable synergy of antibodies to EGFR and chemotherapeutic agents, although the mechanisms of these interactions are unclear. It is of interest that a recent clinical study of a chimaeric monoclonal antibody to EGFR (IMC-225) in patients with advanced CRC, whose disease had progressed after treatment with CPT-11, showed a 17% response as well as a 31% minimal response or stable disease end-point (Saltz *et al.* 2001). This indicates a possible role for growth factor receptor inhibition in CRC in combination with chemotherapy.

Conclusion

Many novel strategies are currently being developed for the treatment of advanced CRC. Apart from novel agents, there is considerable interest in optimising drug delivery to tumour by approaches including liposomal agents or through hepatic arterial infusion. This brief review has not included approaches such as anti-angiogenic molecules, inhibitors of cell adhesion and tumour vaccines, which all show promise. It is clear that many of the new molecules will be cytostatic rather than cytotoxic. Furthermore, there is clearly major scope for combining these agents with cytotoxic agents to synergise activity (Shah & Schwartz 2001). Phase I studies will have to take these factors into account and measure biological end-points either from tumour material or by sophisticated imaging techniques, rather than simply assessing maximum tolerated dose (Gelmon *et al.* 1999). The addition of genomic and proteasomic microarray methodologies will be vital in the development of the translational research networks that will be crucial for the testing and validation of these agents.

References

Adjei AA (2001). Blocking oncogenic ras signaling for cancer therapy. *Journal of the National Cancer Institute* **93**, 1062–1074

Advani R, Saba HI, Tallman MS *et al.* (1999). Treatment of refractory and relapsed acute myelogenous leukemia with combination chemotherapy plus the multidrug resistance modulator PSC 833 (Valspodar). *Blood* **93**, 787–795

Alon U, Barkai N, Notterman DA *et al.* (1999). Broad patterns of gene expression revealed by clustering analysis of tumor and normal colon tissues probed by oligonucleotide arrays. *Proceedings of the National Academy of Sciences of the USA* **96**, 6745–650

Aparicio SA, Caldas C, Ponder B (2000). Does massively parallel transcriptome analysis signify the end of cancer histopathology as we know it? *Genome Biology* **1**(3)

Chung-Faye GA, Kerr DJ, Young LS, Searle PF (2000). Gene therapy strategies for colon cancer. *Molecular Medicine Today* **6**, 82–87

Chiang SY, Burli RW, Benz CC *et al.* (2000). Targeting the ets binding site of the HER2/neu promoter with pyrrole-imidazole polyamides. *Journal of Biological Chemistry* **275**, 24246–24254

Cunningham D, Pyrhonen S, James RD *et al.* (1998). Randomised trial of irinotecan plus supportive care versus supportive care alone after fluorouracil failure for patients with metastatic colorectal cancer. *The Lancet* **352**, 1413–1418

Delaloge S, Yovine A, Taamma A *et al.* (2001). Ecteinascidin-743: a marine-derived compound in advanced, pretreated sarcoma patients—preliminary evidence of activity. *Journal of Clinical Oncology* **19**, 1248–1255

Dervan PB & Burli RW (1999). Sequence-specific DNA recognition by polyamides. *Current Opinions in Chemical Biology* **3**, 688–693

Desai SD, Li TK, Rodriguez-Bauman A *et al.* (2001). Ubiquitin/26S proteasome-mediated degradation of topoisomerase I as a resistance mechanism to camptothecin in tumor cells. *Cancer Research* **61**, 5926–5932

Douillard JY, Cunningham D, Roth AD *et al.* (2000). Irinotecan combined with fluorouracil compared with fluorouracil alone as first-line treatment for metastatic colorectal cancer: a multicentre randomised trial. *The Lancet* **355**, 1041–1047

Fink D, Nebel S, Aebi S *et al.* (1996). The role of DNA mismatch repair in platinum drug resistance. *Cancer Research* **56**, 4881–4886

Fitzgerald GA & Patrono C (2001). Drug therapy: the coxibs, selective inhibitors of cyclooxygenase-2. *New England Journal of Medicine* **345**, 433–442

Gelmon KA, Eisenhauer EA, Harris AL *et al*. (1999). Anticancer agents targeting signaling molecules and cancer cell environment: challenges for drug development? *Journal of the National Cancer Institute* **91**, 1281–1287

Gregson SJ, Howard PW, Hartley JA *et al*. (2001). Design, synthesis, and evaluation of a novel pyrrolobenzodiazepine DNA-interactive agent with highly efficient cross-linking ability and potent cytotoxicity. *Journal of Medicinal Chemistry* **44**, 737–748

Hostein I, Robertson D, DiStefano F *et al*. (2001). Inhibition of signal transduction by the Hsp90 inhibitor 17-allylamino-17-demethoxygeldanamycin results in cytostasis and apoptosis. *Cancer Research* **61**, 4003–4009

Johnston PG, Lenz HJ, Leichman CG *et al*. (1995). Thymidylate synthase gene and protein expression correlate and are associated with response to 5-fluorouracil in human colorectal and gastric tumors. *Cancer Research* **55**, 1407–1412

Kaye SB (1998). Multidrug resistance: clinical relevance in solid tumours and strategies for circumvention. *Current Opinions in Oncology* **10**, S15–S19

Khuri FR, Nemunaitis J, Ganly I *et al*. (2000). A controlled trial of intratumoral ONYX-015, a selectively-replicating adenovirus, in combination with cisplatin and 5-fluorouracil in patients with recurrent head and neck cancer. *Nature Medicine* **6**, 879–885

Kinzler KW & Vogelstein B (1996). Lessons from hereditary colorectal cancer. *Cell* **87**, 159–170

Kirn D (2001). Clinical research results with DL1520 (Onyx-015), a replication-selective adenovirus for the treatment of cancer: what have we learned? Gene Therapy **8**, 89–98

Kudoh K, Ramanna M, Ravatn R *et al*. (2000). Monitoring the expression profiles of doxorubicin-induced and doxorubicin-resistant cancer cells by cDNA microarray. *Cancer Research* **60**, 4161–4166

Mendelsohn J & Baselga J (2000). The EGF receptor family as targets for cancer therapy. *Oncogene* **19**, 6550–6565

Napier MP, Sharma SK, Springer CJ *et al*. (2000).Antibody-directed enzyme pro-drug therapy: efficacy and mechanism of action in colorectal carcinoma. *Clinical Cancer Research* **6**, 765–772

Nevins JR (2001). The Rb/E2F pathway and cancer. *Human Molecular Genetics* **10**, 699–703

Paradiso A, Simone G, Petroni S *et al*. (2000). Thymidylate synthase and p53 primary tumour expression as predictive factors for advanced colorectal cancer patients. *British Journal of Cancer* **82**, 560–567

Saltz L, Rubin M, Hochster H *et al*. (2001). Cetuximab (IMC-C225) plus irinotecan (CPT-11) is active in CPT-11-refractory colorectal cancer (CRC) that expresses epidermal growth factor receptor (EGFR) *Proceedings of the American Society of Clinical Oncology* **20**(7)

Senderowicz AM (2000). Small molecule modulators of cyclin-dependent kinases for cancer therapy. *Oncogene* **19**, 6600–6606

Shah MA & Schwartz GK (2001). Cell cycle-mediated drug resistance: an emerging concept in cancer therapy. *Clinical Cancer Research* **7**, 2168–2181

Strathdee G, MacKean MJ, Illand M, Brown R (1999). A role for methylation of the hMLH1 promoter in loss of hMLH1 expression and drug resistance in ovarian cancer. *Oncogene* **18**, 2335–2341

Steinbach G, Lynch PM., Phillips R. *et al*. (2000). The effect of celecoxib, a cyclooxygenase-2 inhibitor, in familial adenomatous polyposis. *New England Journal of Medicine* **342**, 1946–1952

Thurston DE (1999). Nucleic acid targeting: therapeutic strategies for the 21st century. *British Journal of Cancer* **80**, 65–85

Vaisman A, Varchenko M, Umar A *et al.* (1998). The role of hMLH1, hMSH3, and hMSH6 defects in cisplatin and oxaliplatin resistance: correlation with replicative bypass of platinum-DNA adducts. *Cancer Research* **58**, 3579–3585

Waters JS, Webb A, Cunningham D *et al.* (2000). Phase I clinical and pharmacokinetic study of bcl-2 antisense oligonucleotide therapy in patients with non-Hodgkin's lymphoma. *Journal of Clinical Oncology* **18**, 1812–1823

Webley SD, Francis RJ, Pedley RB *et al.* (2001). Measurement of the critical DNA lesions produced by antibody-directed enzyme prodrug therapy (ADEPT) in vitro, in vivo and in clinical material. *British Journal of Cancer* **84**, 1671–1676

Zewail-Foote M & Hurley LH (1999). Ecteinascidin 743: a minor groove alkylator that bends DNA toward the major groove. *Journal of Medicinal Chemistry* **42**, 2493–2497

PART 3

Rectal cancer

Chapter 9

Total mesorectal excision as a standard surgical procedure: the evidence base for improved clinical outcome

Bill Heald

Introduction

For almost 20 years the concept of total mesorectal excision (TME) has featured in the medical literature (Heald *et al*. 1982; Heald & Ryall 1986; Heald 1987, 1995). It remains, however, the object of ongoing controversy and sometimes of downright antagonism (Isbister 1990, 1998).

This antagonism probably stems from disbelief in the large size of the benefits claimed. There is also an understandable reluctance to accept that local recurrence is largely the result of error that might have been avoided if enough care had been taken. Certainly the impossibility of applying prospective randomised trial techniques to the detail of technical surgery has been a major impediment to its establishment as the new 'gold standard'. No prospective randomised controlled trial (PRCT) has ever been successfully mounted to underpin a complex advance in a surgical technique. Furthermore, significant confusion stems from the development of alternative basic technologies such as laparoscopic surgery. These are amenable to PRCT methods and trials are currently under way. It is important, however, to understand that total mesorectal excision (TME) is an oncological principle that is theoretically achievable by either open or laparoscopic methods; these trials will add nothing to the most crucial controversy – the detail of the excision of the tumour.

Total mesorectal excision is a system of cancer management that defines the block of tissue to be excised and describes the surgical detail of how this is to be achieved. It is now more readily comprehended by non-surgeons because of the development by specialised magnetic resonance imaging (MRI) radiologists of images that are far superior to anything so far achievable (Figures 9.1 and 9.2). These demonstrate, for the first time, the contours of the mesorectum and the distribution of the cancer within it. They will almost certainly in the future provide a rational basis for selecting those cases for radiotherapy or chemoradiotherapy, where the mesorectal margin is in danger of being breached during surgery.

The TME concept can be extended now to embrace phased-array-coil 3-mm slice (high-quality) MRI, detailed precision surgery and detailed audit of the specimen after removal. TME comprises five basic principles:

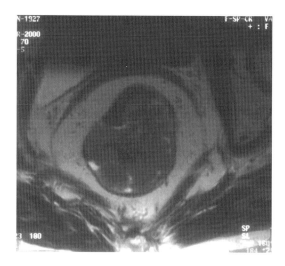

Figure 9.1 Female patient: lumen filled with villous tumour with malignant change but no penetration through into the mesorectal fat. (Reproduced with the kind permission of Dr Delia Peppercorn, The North Hampshire Hospital.)

1. Perimesorectal 'Holy Plane' sharp dissection with diathermy and scissors under direct vision.
2. Specimen-oriented surgery and histopathology, of which the objective is an intact mesorectum with no tearing of the surface and no circumferential margin involvement (CMI) – naked eye or microscopic. Quirke-style pathology audit for CMI as the principal outcome measure confirms the success or failure of the surgery.
3. Recognition and preservation of the autonomic nerve plexus, on which sexual and bladder function depend.
4. A major increase in anal preservation and reduction in the number of permanent colostomies.
5. Stapled low pelvic reconstruction, usually using the Moran triple stapling technique plus a short colon pouch anastomosed to low rectum or anal canal (Moran *et al.* 1994).

In August 1998, Professor John MacFarlane, from the University of British Columbia, published the second set of Basingstoke data from his independent audit of the results in Basingstoke. This comprised a personal series of 519 consecutive surgical cases with adenocarcinoma treated for cure or palliation (Heald *et al.* 1998). The largest group was 465 anterior resections (ARs) with low stapled anastomosis (407 TME), 37 abdominoperineal (AP) resections, 10 Hartmann resections, 4 local excisions and 3 laparotomy only. Preoperative radiotherapy was used in 49 cases (7 AP, 38 AR, 3 Hartmann, 1 laparotomy). Cancer-specific survival (CSS) rate of all

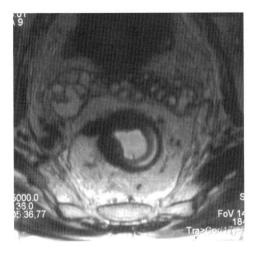

Figure 9.2 Male patient: direct invasion of mesorectal fat on right. (Reproduced with the kind permission of Dr Delia Peppercorn, The North Hampshire Hospital.)

surgically treated cases is 68% at 5 years and 66% at 10 years. There is a 6% local recurrence (LR) rate at 5 years (2–10% at 95% confidence interval [95%CI]), 8% at 10 years (2–14% at 95%CI). In 405 'curative' resections the LR rate is 3% and 4% and the CSS rate 80% and 78% at 5 years and 10 years, respectively. All patients were followed regularly until death. The principal risk factors for recurrence include the necessity to perform AP as opposed to AR (for LR), Dukes' stage (for CSS) and extramural vascular invasion (EVI) (for LR and CSS).

Substantial improvements on all previously published, comprehensive, unselected series now appear confirmed beyond all doubts by these data. In addition, it becomes clear that low LR rates have a substantial effect on overall survival, i.e. that many LRs after conventional surgery are the result of regrowth of local mesorectal residues, which were the only disease present at the time of surgery. Thus local control equates with cure in such cases and better local control with more cures.

Total mesorectal excision and precise perimesorectal plane dissection are being introduced in all the major countries of Europe. Increasingly, the specimen is being audited by the detailed histopathology of Quirke and Dixon (1998). In a trial under way in the Netherlands, the CMI is being carefully monitored as a principal surgical outcome, so that a real and immediate quality control routine can be introduced. The most significant new evidence comes from a joint publication from the Stockholm Colorectal Cancer Group and the Basingstoke Bowel Cancer Research Project. In *The Lancet* in July 2000 the first published report appeared, showing a major impact of a teaching programme on cancer outcomes in an entire population. Both the permanent colostomy rate and the local recurrence rate have been more than halved for the entire population of Stockholm County (Lehander *et al.* 2000).

A major publication is awaited from Norway (Soreide, unpublished data) where a similar teaching programme was introduced while a PRCT of monitored and supervised TME with or without short course radiotherapy has now closed in the Netherlands with 800 patients in each arm. A further study is well advanced in Denmark. Individual series such as those already published in the USA by Enker and in New Zealand by Hill show strikingly similar results to those in Basingstoke. Certainly the initial widespread dismissal of the early Basingstoke results with single figure local recurrence rates are set aside by others achieving exactly the same. In all the individual surgeon series, there is a significant improvement on the multi-surgeon series, as would be anticipated for a technique that is technically demanding and challenging.

It is now generally accepted in Europe and in many parts of the world that more precise surgery directed towards mesorectal excision is the principal determinant of outcome and the principal hope for improvement. The author has undertaken 150 television workshop demonstration operations in 22 countries. TME has become the national standard in Norway, Sweden, Denmark and the Netherlands. In the larger countries – Germany, France and the UK – official guidelines support the TME concept. In Germany major studies are ongoing to introduce it and even to embrace the specialisation and audit routines necessary to eliminate the surgeon variability that Hermanek *et al.* (1995) has so ably demonstrated.

Conclusion

Until the TME controversy, almost nothing was published about dissection around a rectal cancer. An arbitrary 5-cm distal margin along the muscle tube and the relevance or irrelevance of the internal iliac nodes had provoked some lingering controversy. Ten years ago local recurrence rates between 25% and 50% were standard, and recurrence within the pelvis was by far the most common pattern. The early claims from Basingstoke of single figure local recurrence rates by TME were complemented by reports from Leeds which showed a high positive predictive value of CMI LR (Quirke & Dixon 1998). What has been difficult for many to comprehend is that this high predictive value applies only to series where the local recurrence rate is high, e.g. in Leeds at the time of the first CMI publication the overall local recurrence rate was 36%, whereas CMI was a much poorer predictor in Guildford where TME surgery was delivering a much lower LR rate (Editorial 1990). Reports also appeared of wide variations in results between surgeons. The fact that three-quarters of the Leeds LRs had been predicted by CMI reflected a key reality, which went largely unnoticed; most of these CMI cases could have been avoided by the wider circumferential clearance afforded by TME. Thus the lower the local recurrence rate in any given series, the less good a predictor CMI becomes, although it remains a predictor of cancer death.

The real importance of CMI is, however, that it provides a key audit tool for better surgery. It is axiomatic that the margins of a cancer specimen must be clear of cancer: low CMI rates reflect 'better' surgery and are an end in themselves; if TME surgeons deliver lower CMI rates then this is a self-evident benefit.

Most advances now seem to be initiated by developments in technology. If the scientific basis for the TME operation can be improved the outcomes are likely to improve and more meaningful trials established in the future, based on measurable criteria. The phased-array-coil fine-slice MRI, in the hands of a suitably trained radiologist, is one such seminal step forward. This walk-in non-invasive investigation, with no bowel preparation, can provide preoperatively three-dimensional detail of the distribution of cancer within the defined block of tissue to be excised – the mesorectum. Thus, tumour height, anteroposterior position and proximity to the mesorectal margin can all be objectively recorded and decisions about radiotherapy and chemotherapy made before the surgery date is set. TME can be taught to surgeons and their success in reaching the defined objective measured by the histopathologist. Those relatively few rectal cancers where the whole mesorectum does not need to be removed (e.g. those above around 12 cm sigmoidoscopically) will be readily defined. What is a safe margin will become an objective measurement instead of a clinical guess. The observational studies, and personal series, of the past will become more precise.

Those aspects of management amenable to prospective and randomised controlled study, such as radiotherapy and chemotherapy, will be the object of trials, whereas the surgical detail will be accurately analysed by histopathological audit. In all these ways rectal cancer can indeed be a paradigm for the management of all solid tumours.

References

Editorial (1990). Breaching the mesorectum. *The Lancet* **335**, 1067–1068

Heald RJ, Husband EM, Ryall RDH (1982). The mesorectum is rectal cancer surgery – the clue to pelvic recurrence? *British Journal of Surgery* **69**, 613–616

Heald RJ & Ryall RDH (1986). Recurrence and survival after total mesorectal excision for rectal cancer. *The Lancet* **i**, 1479–1482

Heald RJ, Moran BJ, Ryall RDH, Sexton R, MacFarlane JK (1998). Rectal Cancer. The Basingstoke Experience of Total Mesorectal Excision, 1978–1997. *Archives of Surgery* **133**, 894–898

Heald RJ (1995). Total mesorectal excision is optimal surgery for rectal cancer: a Scandinavian consensus. Leading article *British Journal of Surgery* **82**, 1297–1299

Heald RJ (1997). Total mesorectal excision: history and anatomy of an operation. In Soreide O, Norstein J, eds, *Rectal Cancer Surgery: Optimisation – standardisation – documentation*. Berlin: Springer-Verlag, pp 203–219

Hermanek P, Wiebelt H, Staimmer D, Riedl S (1995). Prognostic factors of rectum carcinoma – experience of the German Multicenter Study SGCRC German Study Group Colo-Rectal Carcinoma. *Tumori* **8**(suppl 3), 60–64

Isbister WH (1990). Basingstoke revisited. *Australia and New Zealand Journal of Surgery* **60**, 243–246

Isbister WH (1998). Food for thought – Basingstoke revisited again. *Australia and New Zealand Journal of Surgery* in press

Lehander Martling A, Holm T *et al.* (2000). Effect of a surgical training programme on outcome of rectal cancer in the County of Stockholm. *The Lancet* **356**, 93–96

Moran BJ, Docherty A, Finnis D (1994). Novel stapling technique to facilitate low anterior resection for rectal cancer. *British Journal of Surgery* **81**, 1230

Quirke P & Dixon MF (1998). The prediction of local recurrence of rectal adenocarcinoma by histopathological examination. *International Journal of Colorectal Disease* **3**, 127–131

Local staging of rectal cancer: the clinical effectiveness of high-resolution MRI

Gina Brown and Ceri J Phillips

Local staging of rectal cancer

The purpose of a good staging technique is to be able to separate patients into distinct prognostic groups. This is of importance in defining the subgroups of patients who have different risks of recurrence and who could be treated more or less intensively. The need for standardised and thorough reporting of rectal cancer surgical specimens has led to the introduction of standardised pathology reporting (Bull *et al.* 1997). The minimum dataset and the more detailed UKCCCR clinicopathological reporting of colorectal cancer takes into account the many important prognostic factors that may govern survival. Clearly, preoperative knowledge of these factors is also important given the potential of preoperative therapy to downstage tumours. The important prognostic factors are summarised below and the potential role of MRI in demonstrating this is illustrated.

Patterns of spread

When rectal tumours invade through the bowel wall into perirectal fat, they commonly do so with a well-circumscribed margin. In 25% of cases, however, the pattern of spread is infiltrative with ill-defined borders. The pattern of spread in the latter has been shown to worsen prognosis (Grinnell 1939; Spratt & Spjut 1967; Jass *et al.* 1986). Conversely, the presence of an inflammatory response at the advancing margin of the tumour has been observed as a favourable prognostic feature (Jass *et al.* 1986). Regardless of differentiation, colorectal tumours, unlike upper gastrointestinal tumours, rarely show submucous or intramural spread beyond their macroscopic borders. This characteristic is important in the surgical planning of distal resection margins (Hughes *et al.* 1983; Madsen & Christiansen 1986; Andreola *et al.* 1997) and current evidence based on data examining intramural spread suggests that a 1-cm distal clearance is sufficient to ensure complete distal clearance of the tumour.

Mucinous tumours

Mucinous tumours form a distinct morphological subgroup characterised by their watery appearance resulting from secretion of mucus by the tumour cells, and account for 10% of carcinomas of the large intestine. These tumours appear to represent a poor prognostic subgroup, which is thought to relate to their propensity to infiltrate diffusely and, unlike non-mucinous tumours, these may spread intramurally (Madsen & Christiansen 1986; Sidoni *et al.* 1991) (Figures 10.1–10.3).

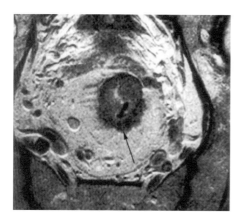
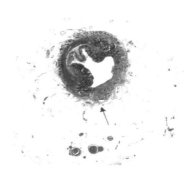

Figure 10.1 Well-defined border (MR image with histological correlation). Axial high-resolution T2-weighted image and corresponding whole-mount section (haematoxylin and eosin [H&E] stained). The advancing edge of the tumour (arrow) has a well-circumscribed margin with a sharp border between the advancing edge of tumour and perirectal fat. This is the most common pattern of tumour spread.

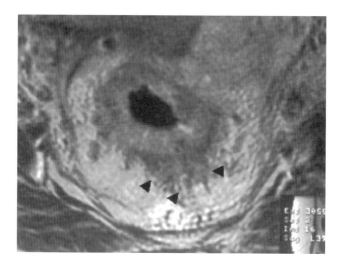

Figure 10.2 Infiltrative spread of tumour (high-resolution axial MRI). Axial T2-weighted FSE image shows nodular extension (arrow heads) of tumour into perirectal fat producing an ill-defined tumour border at the advancing margin.

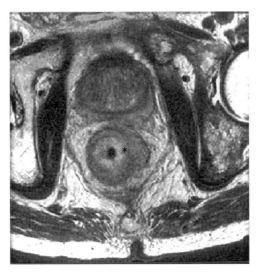

Figure 10.3 Mucinous tumours are characterised by very high signal intensity (high water content) tumour (*) which infiltrated bowel wall without destroying the boundaries between individual layers – resulting in accentuation or thickening of the bowel wall layers.

Circumferential resection margin

In 1982, the importance of involvement of the lateral circumferential margin by tumour and its relationship to local recurrence were prospectively investigated (Quirke *et al*. 1986). The risk of local recurrence in circumferential resection margin (CRM)-positive patients was significantly higher than in CRM-negative patients and, compared with CRM-negative patients, the risk of death was three times higher. Moreover, CRM-positive patients had only a 15% 5-year survival rate. CRM involvement became a powerful predictor of local recurrence and an important new addition to the pathological staging of rectal cancer.

In the initial study, each tumour was embedded in its entirety with preparation of multiple whole-mount blocks. Quirke later showed that visual inspection of the macroscopic slices was sufficient to select sections with suspected CRM involvement (Quirke & Dixon 1988; Adam *et al*. 1994). This proved to be robust in practice and reproducible in other histopathology institutions (de Haas-Kock *et al*. 1996) (Figure 10.4).

Spread beyond the peritoneal membrane

Local peritoneal involvement was detected in 25.8% (54 of 209) of cases. This is defined as perforation of the peritoneal membrane by tumour, and the consequent spillage of tumour cells is presumed to result in both local recurrence and transcoelomic dissemination. This was an independent prognostic factor and predicted for local recurrence after surgery for upper and middle rectal cancer (Shepherd *et al.* 1995) (Figure 10.5).

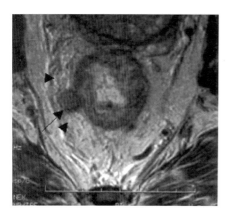
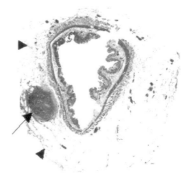

Figure 10.4 Positive CRM on MRI and histology. An extramural tumour deposit above the level of the intramural tumour (arrow) abuts the mesorectal fascia (arrow heads). If tumour lies within 1 mm of the mesorectal fascia, this predicts for positive circumferential resection margin (CRM) status. Subsequent total mesorectal excision specimen shows tumour at the margin.

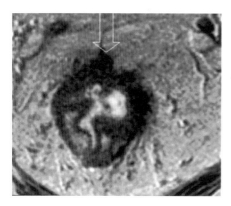
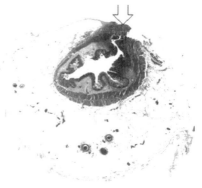

Figure 10.5 MRI and histology sections showing T4 infiltration. Nodular extension of tumour into the peritoneal reflection (arrow) is demonstrated on both preoperative MRI and histology sections.

Lymph node spread

The presence of lymph node metastases in the resected specimen worsens prognosis and this effect is most pronounced when four or more nodes are affected. However, Rich *et al.* (1983) observed that the incidence of local failure for tumours without lymph node metastasis was 17% in tumours with only microscopic extension through the wall. Similarly, in tumours with positive lymph nodes, local failure was lower in tumours confined to the wall or with only microscopic extension, compared with tumours with extensive spread through the wall. Significant differences in survival are observed when Dukes' C cases are subdivided according to depth of tumour penetration as proposed by Astler and Coller and designated as C1 and C2 (Fisher *et al.* 1989). The prognostic advantage of Astler–Coller C1 over Astler–Coller C2 status has also been confirmed by Jass and Love (1989), who showed that spread was an important prognostic variable for survival. In this study, estimated 5-year survival rate for Astler–Coller C1 cases was just below 80% and similar to Astler–Coller stage B2 (Dukes' B) cases.

For one, 2–5, 6–10 and more than 10 affected nodes the 5-year survival rates were 63.6%, 36.1%, 21.9% and 2.1%, respectively (Dukes & Bussey 1958). This observation was reaffirmed (Wolmark *et al.* 1984; Jass *et al.* 1986; Moran *et al.* 1992) illustrating the importance of ensuring adequate node sampling through meticulous lymph node dissection (Andreola *et al.* 1997) (Figure 10.6).

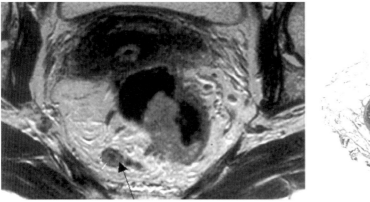
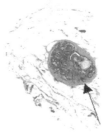

Figure 10.6 Node containing tumour on MRI with corresponding histology section. A mixed signal intensity node is defined as abnormal if it contains mixed signal intensity or has irregular borders. In this case, a mixed signal intensity deposit (arrow) predicted corresponded to a tumour-containing node.

Venous spread

Spread into thick-walled extramural veins carries a very poor prognosis. In one series, the corrected 5-year survival rate for Dukes' stage C patients with invasion of thick-walled veins was only 8% and invasion of extramural veins was associated with a low 5-year survival rate of 33% (Talbot *et al*. 1981). Others have reaffirmed this observation (Horn *et al*. 1990, 1991; Bokey *et al*. 1999). Moreover, in models using step-wise selection of prognostic indicators, extramural venous invasion has been shown to retain independent prognostic significance (Bokey *et al*. 1999; Harrison *et al*. 1994) (Figure 10.7).

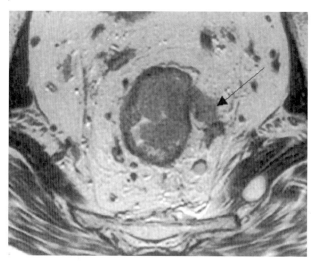

Figure 10.7 There is a serpiginous extension of tumour into perirectal fat (arrow) which corresponded to thick-walled extramural venous invasion.

The extent of local spread

Dukes' (1932) paper highlighted the importance of extent of extramural spread in the prediction of local recurrence as well as survival. Survival figures for Dukes' B cases were 89.7% for slight spread, 80% for moderate spread and 57% for extensive spread. The measurement is taken from the outer edge of the longitudinal muscle layer. Importantly, Dukes also observed that, once spread beyond the bowel wall occurs, the incidence of lymph node invasion increases, rising from 14.2% in tumours confined to the bowel wall to 43.2% in those tumours extending beyond the bowel wall.

In 1979, an international staging system was adopted based on a TNM classification whereby local spread of the primary tumour is denoted by T, regional lymph nodes as N and metastases as M. The system was introduced to overcome confusion between existing staging classifications (namely Dukes and Astler–Coller). The TNM classification allowed a clinical staging based on digital rectal examination and computed tomography (CT) examination findings to be incorporated (denoted by the prefix c, i.e. cTNM) and considered with the pathologist's assessment of TNM stage (denoted by the prefix p, i.e. pTNM). The TNM classification for colorectal cancer has since been modified further (Table 10.1) and the most recent edition was published in 1997 (Sobin & Wittekind 1997). In 1993, an optional modification of the TNM system (Table 10.2) was proposed to take into account the importance of extramural spread as a means of distinguishing between an otherwise heterogeneous group of T3 tumours and also included a separate classification of T4 tumours to distinguish between peritoneal perforation (pT4b) and invasion of adjacent pelvic structures (pT4a) (Hermanek *et al.* 1993). The advantages of telescoping were to allow the collection of additional important prognostic data without altering the definitions of the existing TNM categories. Hermanek also noted the importance of incorporating important and independent prognostic factors while retaining an intact TNM system, and postulated that a future sophisticated prognostic index incorporating such data may be used to assign patients to various prognostic groups. In doing so, this could enable the better design of future trials by appropriate stratification based on all relevant prognostic factors. The value of MRI in accurately measuring extramural depth has already been shown (Brown *et al.* 1999) and it may be appropriate to incorporate such measurements in future staging systems and clinical trials.

Clinical effectiveness of preoperative staging in rectal cancer: MRI, digital rectal examination or endoluminal ultrasonography

Local recurrence is a major cause of morbidity and mortality in rectal cancer, occurring in up to 50% of cases (Frykholm *et al.* 1995). Although meticulous surgical technique, as exemplified by total mesorectal excision (TME), has improved survival by reducing local recurrences in selected patients (Heald 1995; Carlsen *et al.* 1998; Heald *et al.* 1998), it is unclear whether these results will be generalisable. Preoperative neoadjuvant radiotherapy and chemoradiotherapy regimens also promise to improve survival (Swedish Rectal Cancer Trial 1997; Marsh *et al.* 1994; Dahlberg *et al.* 1998; Pahlman 1998), but their success needs to be tempered by the inevitable morbidity associated with such treatments (Dahlberg *et al.* 1998). Ideally, the intensity of preoperative treatment needs to be tailored to the local disease stage. Among the most important factors affecting local recurrence are the degree of tumour penetration through the bowel wall at the time of surgery and its relationship to the CRMs (Chung *et al.* 1983; Adam *et al.* 1994). An accurate method of assessing these features, and of tumour stage in general, preoperatively in all rectal cancer patients could therefore allow optimal selection for a range of treatment strategies.

Numerous studies have shown endoluminal ultrasonography (EUS) to be superior to CT in the local staging of rectal tumours (Beynon *et al.* 1989; Mehta *et al.* 1994; Kim *et al.* 1999). Digital rectal examination (DRE) combined with EUS is currently

Table 10.1 The TNM classification of rectal cancer (Sobin & Wittekind 1997)

TNM definitions

Primary tumour (T)

TX:	Primary tumour cannot be assessed
T0:	No evidence of primary tumour
Tis:	Carcinoma *in situ*: intraepithelial or invasion of the lamina propria[a]
T1:	Tumour invades submucosa
T2:	Tumour invades muscularis propria
T3:	Tumour invades through the muscularis propria into the subserosa, or into non-peritonealised pericolic or perirectal tissues
T4:	Tumour directly invades other organs or structures, and/or perforates visceral peritoneum[b]

Regional lymph nodes (N)

NX:	Regional nodes cannot be assessed
N0:	No regional lymph node metastasis
N1:	Metastasis in one to three regional lymph nodes
N2:	Metastasis in four or more regional lymph nodes

Distant metastasis (M)

MX:	Distant metastasis cannot be assessed
M0:	No distant metastasis
M1:	Distant metastasis

A tumour nodule > 3 mm in diameter in the perirectal or pericolic fat without histological evidence of a residual node in the nodule is classified as regional perirectal or pericolic lymph node metastasis.

A tumour nodule ≤ 3 mm in diameter is classified in the T category as a non-contiguous extension, i.e. T3.

[a]This includes cancer cells confined within the glandular basement membrane (intraepithelial) or lamina propria (intramucosal) with no extension through the muscularis mucosae into the submucosa.

[b]Direct invasion in T4 includes invasion of other segments of the colorectum by way of the serosa, e.g. invasion of the sigmoid colon by a carcinoma of the caecum.

recommended as the staging method of choice (Royal College of Surgeons and the Association of Coloproctology of Great Britain and Ireland 1996). Unfortunately, up to 20% of patients presenting with rectal cancer cannot be evaluated by EUS as a result of luminal narrowing by bulky or stricturing tumours and high rectal tumours cannot be fully assessed by DRE (Lindmark *et al.* 1994). Early studies assessing magnetic resonance imaging (MRI) have also been disappointing; poor spatial

Table 10.2 Proposals for further development of the TNM system: 'telescopic ramifications'

T stage	Definition
pT3	According to histologically measured perimuscular invasion
pT3a (minimal)	< 1 mm
pT3b (slight)	1–5 mm
pT3c (moderate)	5–15 mm
pT3d (extensive)	>15 mm
pT4	
pT4a	Invasion of adjacent organs or structures
pT4b	Perforation of visceral peritoneum

resolution and an inability to demonstrate the bowel wall layers have resulted in overstaging (Kusunoki *et al.* 1994; McNicholas *et al.* 1994; Zerhouni *et al.* 1994). Endorectal MRI, while offering superior spatial resolution, suffers the same limitations as other endoluminal techniques (Schnall *et al.* 1994). Two recent studies (Urban *et al.* 2000; Wallengren *et al.* 2000) recommend the use of contrast agents with MRI in order to identify the intraluminal portion of the tumour. The technique adds little to the assessment of the extramural component of tumour that governs selection for preoperative. Recently, studies have compared EUS and MRI (Blomqvist *et al.* 2000; Gualdi *et al.* 2000; Maldjian *et al.* 2000). Some of these studies used only an endorectal MRI technique, which is an invasive procedure that cannot be used in at least 20% of patients. Of the studies that have evaluated pelvic phase array or body coil MRI, none has employed the high-resolution technique described or considered the clinically important separation of T3 tumours with favourable or unfavourable prognosis.

Using a high-resolution technique, thin-slice MRI can be used to measure the depth of extramural spread accurately, with good correlation with corresponding pathology measurements in resection specimens (Brown *et al.* 1999). The technique has the advantages of being non-invasive; employing a short imaging time (30–40 minutes), and it can be performed using standard software on a 1.5-T field strength magnet. A recent study (Beets-Tan *et al.* 2000) using a similar high-resolution technique showed correlation between the MRI measurement of tumour distance to the CRM and the corresponding histological measurement.

Rationale for the use of MRI

In patients who are unlikely to be cured by surgery alone, preoperative neoadjuvant therapy is of potential value in tumour downstaging. However, there is little evidence to suggest that intensive preoperative combined modality therapy benefits patients with early stage disease. It is clear that the role of preoperative staging is to distinguish between tumours that have favourable and unfavourable prognostic features.

Numerous pathological studies have clarified these prognostic features and a possible rationale for therapy is summarised in Figure 10.8.

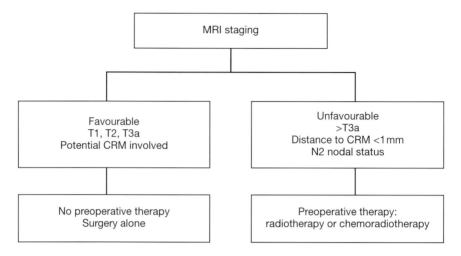

Figure 10.8 Model treatment pathway following preoperative staging by MRI. MRI allows preoperative identification of important prognostic factors permitting identification of patients with tumours who can be cured by surgery alone and patients at risk of local recurrence or poor survival who may benefit from preoperative therapy.

Evaluation of clinical effectiveness

In a recent study, the agreement for the extent of extramural spread and tumour involvement of the CRM among DRE, EUS and MRI, with the pathology gold standard, assesses the ability of these preoperative staging methods to distinguish favourable from unfavourable tumours (Brown *et al.* 2000). Both DRE and EUS assessment show poor agreement with pathology and DRE understaged 29% of patients (95% confidence interval [95%CI] 15.8–41.3%). MRI had a clear advantage in sensitivity over EUS (MRI and EUS, $\Delta = 0.241$, 95%CI +0.015–0.440) and a slight advantage in specificity (MRI and EUS, $\Delta = 0.077$ 95%CI, +0.096–0.252).

Agreement between MRI and pathology in distinguishing favourable from unfavourable tumours was very good at 0.86 ($\kappa = 0.71$, 95%CI 0.55–0.83). The main limitation of MRI is in the distinction between T1 and T2 tumours and between T2 tumours and tumours with < 1 mm spread into perirectal fat. EUS was less successful in distinguishing favourable from unfavourable tumours with an agreement of 0.69 ($\kappa = 0.38$, 95%CI 0.12–0.59), largely as a result of problems in assessing upper rectal lesions. Patients with favourable tumours were overstaged by EUS as having extramural tumour extension of > 5 mm whereas many patients with unfavourable tumours were understaged. DRE assessment of tumour mobility was poor at distinguishing favourable from unfavourable tumours. In the same study, 25% of rectal tumours were too high to assess digitally and 79% of these were in the unfavourable group. Conversely, only 7% of locally advanced pathological stage tumours (pT4 or extramural spread > 15 mm) was said to be fixed. Conversely, of the eight clinically fixed tumours, only one was locally extensive on pathology.

With regard to CRM involvement, this correlated poorly with tethering or fixity on DRE. On the other hand, MRI assessment was good at predicting this: 77% of tumours with predicted CRM positivity on MRI were confirmed by pathology. In the remaining patients, MRI failed to identify pathological CRM involvement as a result of microscopic deposits in lymph nodes at the CRM, and not tumour in continuity with the primary lesion.

Economic implications

The extent to which staging methods can distinguish between favourable and unfavourable tumours has obvious implications for neoadjuvant therapy and surgical procedures, and the resulting resource implications. The consequence of understaging tumours is the likelihood of recurrence increases, with relatively high costs of treatment involved (Neymark & Adriaenssen 1999), although for tumours that are overstaged treatment is provided that is both unnecessary and expensive.

A short course of radiotherapy is likely to cost in the region of £400 and long-course radiotherapy around £2,000, whereas the resource implications of understaging are likely to be around £5,000 (based on Neymark & Adriaenssen, 1999, and adjusted for a 50% probability of recurrence).

The cost of an MRI varies between centres, but the greater capacity of MRI to produce accurate staging of rectal tumours means that the costs associated with unsuccessful and inaccurate staging, which exist with DRE and EUS, exceed the difference in the costs of procedure between EUS and MRI. In reality the extent of the difference in staging accuracy is likely to result in significant cost savings from using MRI as the staging modality for rectal cancer. It does not therefore require a significant difference in the relative staging accuracy to offset the difference in procedure costs between MRI and EUS.

Discussion

When meticulous histopathological assessment of tumour staging is used as a rigorous gold standard, the benefits of thin-slice, T2-weighted, high-resolution MRI are clearly demonstrated. When compared with other modalities for staging rectal cancer preoperatively, the technique is not only more accurate, but non-invasive and therefore acceptable to virtually all patients. The increased accuracy translates into better patient selection for neoadjuvant therapy and improved clinical effectiveness as well as potential overall cost savings. Moreover, the MR images allow visualisation of the whole of the tumour, its anatomical disposition in any plane extramurally and its relationship to the CRM, all of which greatly assist the planning of any preoperative radiotherapy and the surgical resection itself.

The accuracy of preoperative staging of extramural features of the tumour has been the main focus because this has the greatest influence on treatment selection for the majority of patients presenting with rectal cancer who have T3 lesions. Although there is growing evidence that preoperative radiotherapy and TME have an additive (Holm *et al.* 1997) effect on improvement of local recurrence rates, it is becoming clear that preoperative radiotherapy for 'good' prognosis patients is overtreatment that wastes resources and leads to significant morbidity (Dahlberg *et al.* 1998). Many studies have shown that the depth of extramural invasion and CRM involvement are independent markers of poor prognosis (Jass & Love *al.* 1989; Cawthorn *et al.* 1990) and selection for neoadjuvant therapy needs to be based on these. MRI performs particularly well over other modalities in the assessment of these parameters: our previous studies have validated the technique for accuracy of depth of extramural spread and the present study also demonstrates its ability to predict CRM involvement (Brown *et al.* 1999). By contrast, DRE (which depends on the subjective appreciation of tumour mobility or fixity) performs poorly, understaging nearly 30% of cases. EUS tends to overestimate tumour depth (as a result of the obliquity of the probe in relation to the lesion and difficulty in separating peritumoral inflammation or fibrosis from true tumour) and cannot visualise the mesorectal fascia that represents the CRM. Both techniques are able to assess discontinuous mesorectal tumour deposits that might govern operability for cure, and both are invasive, potentially painful modalities that cannot be applied to all patients for technical reasons.

Through very meticulous pathological correlation, a number of new criteria have been developed by which to stage patients. One of the important findings is that T2 weighting with high resolution will depict tumour as different signal intensity when compared with bowel wall and perirectal fat. The images produced have a high degree of concordance with the gross histological sections, and established histological methods of staging tumour have directly contributed to the development of MR image analysis criteria. The performance of EUS reported recently (Brown *et al.* 2000) showed a far lower accuracy in this study than in previous reports. This may relate to inclusion of all rectal cancer patients regardless of height from the anal sphincter. Previous studies evaluating EUS have tended to exclude higher rectal tumours. The inaccuracy of EUS in nodal staging relates to the high percentage of positive nodes that were < 5 mm in diameter and that were also above the level of the tumour. The poor performance of EUS in staging nodes has been demonstrated in a study using node-wise correlation (Spinelli *et al.* 1999), confirming the inability of EUS to detect positive nodes < 5 mm in diameter. Previous EUS studies have not incorporated measurements of extramural depth in analysis and the obliquity of the probe with respect to the tumour, as well as lack of clear demonstration of the outer longitudinal muscle coat, contributed to inaccurate measurements of extramural depth. These limitations have been noted by others (Hulsmans *et al*. 1994; Akasu *et al*. 1997). The majority of published EUS papers demonstrate accuracies in excess of 90% for T staging; such series, however, have a disproportionately high percentage of early T1 and T2 tumours (up to 60% in some series) (Rifkin & Marks 1985; Feifel *et al*. 1987; Katsura *et al*. 1992). Pathology data (Jass 1986; Shepherd *et al*. 1995) suggest that less than 15% of rectal tumours are confined to bowel wall at presentation. Thus, lack of patient selection may account for the relatively poor performance of EUS at T staging. Indeed, MRI appeared to be poor at separating T1 from T2 tumours and in distinguishing sessile or polypoid adenomas from T1 adenocarcinomas, whereas EUS has been shown to be a robust technique for staging early lesions (Katsura *et al*. 1992). Thus, MRI cannot be recommended as a technique for selecting patients for local excision. However, the rationale for local removal of early tumours but not its draining lymph nodes is controversial (Goldstein & Hart 1999; Garcia-Aguilar *et al*. 2000*)*.

Any analysis of clinical effectiveness and cost-effectiveness in the preoperative staging of rectal cancer is complex because there is at present no single agreed treatment protocol. MRI shows clear-cut clinical benefits and significant cost savings over the traditional method using combined DRE and EUS, in terms of correct allocation of patients to treatment groups for radiotherapy and/or chemotherapy. Thus, the advantages of preoperative high-resolution MRI in selecting appropriate patients for neoadjuvant therapy justify its routine use in the local staging of rectal cancer patients.

Conclusion

Despite aggressive surgery, local recurrence remains the dominant pattern of failure. The key to reducing local recurrence lies in aggressive primary treatment. In patients who are unlikely to be cured by surgery alone, preoperative neoadjuvant therapy is of potential value in tumour downstaging. An assessment of tumour regression, and thus assessment of the efficacy of preoperative therapy in downstaging, is not possible without accurate and thorough pre-treatment documentation of tumour stage incorporating the known pathological prognostic variables.

The pathological staging of tumours into distinct prognostic groups relies exclusively on static morphological features. Clearly, the identification of such factors in the postoperative patient gives useful prognostic information about likelihood of survival, but may be too late to influence survival substantially. It is of great importance therefore to identify these factors preoperatively in order to optimise preoperative therapy and the primary surgical procedure.

*References*_____

Adam IJ, Mohamdee MO, Martin IG *et al*. (1994). The role of circumferential margin involvement in the local recurrence of rectal cancer. *The Lancet* **344**, 707–711

Akasu T, Sugihara K, Moriya Y, Fujita S (1997). Limitations and pitfalls of transrectal ultrasonography for staging of rectal cancer. *Diseases of the Colon & Rectum* **40**, S10–15

Andreola S, Leo E, Belli F *et al.* (1997). Distal intramural spread in adenocarcinoma of the lower third of the rectum treated with total rectal resection and coloanal anastomosis. *Diseases of the Colon & Rectum* **40**(1), 25–29

Beets-Tan RG, Beets GL, Borstlap AC *et al.* (2000). Preoperative assessment of local tumor extent in advanced rectal cancer: CT or high-resolution MRI? *Abdominal Imaging* **25**, 533–541

Beynon J, Mortensen NJ, Foy DM, Channer JL, Rigby H, Virjee J (1989). Preoperative assessment of mesorectal lymph node involvement in rectal cancer. *British Journal of Surgery* **76**, 276–279

Blomqvist L, Machado M, Rubio C *et al.* (2000). Rectal tumour staging: MR imaging using pelvic phased-array and endorectal coils vs endoscopic ultrasonography. *European Radiology* **10**, 653–660

Bokey EL, Ojerskog B, Chapuis PH, Dent OF, Newland RC, Sinclair G (1999). Local recurrence after curative excision of the rectum for cancer without adjuvant therapy: role of total anatomical dissection. *British Journal of Surgery* **86**, 1164–1170

Brown G, Richards CJ, Newcombe RG *et al.* (1999). Rectal carcinoma: thin section MR imaging for staging in 28 patients. *Radiology* **211**, 215–222

Brown G, Williams GT, Phillips CJ *et al.* (2000). Rectal cancer staging using thin-slice MRI compared with EUS(endorectal ultrasound) in 100 patients. *Radiology* **217**, 231

Bull AD, Biffin AH, Mella J *et al.* (1997). Colorectal cancer pathology reporting: a regional audit. *Journal of Clinical Pathology* **50**, 138–142

Carlsen E, Schlichting E, Guldvog I, Johnson E, Heald RJ (1998). Effect of the introduction of total mesorectal excision for the treatment of rectal cancer. *British Journal of Surgery* **85**, 526–529

Cawthorn SJ, Parums DV, Gibbs NM *et al.* (1990). Extent of mesorectal spread and involvement of lateral resection margin as prognostic factors after surgery for rectal cancer. *The Lancet* **335**, 1055–1059

Chung CK, Stryker JA, Demuth WE (1983). Patterns of failure following surgery alone for colorectal carcinoma. *Journal of Surgical Oncology* **22**, 65–70

Dahlberg M, Glimelius B, Graf W, Pahlman L (1998). Preoperative irradiation affects functional results after surgery for rectal cancer: results from a randomized study. *Diseases of the Colon & Rectum* **41**, 543–549; discussion 549–551

de Haas-Kock DF, Baeten CG, Jager JJ *et al.* (1996). Prognostic significance of radial margins of clearance in rectal cancer [see comments]. *British Journal of Surgery* **83**, 781–785

Dukes CE (1932) The classification of cancer of the rectum. *Journal of Pathology and Bacteriology* **35**, 323

Dukes CE & Bussey (1958). The spread of cancer and its effect on prognosis. *British Journal of Cancer* **12**, 309–320

Feifel G, Hildebrandt U *et al.* (1987). Assessment of depth of invasion in rectal cancer by endosonography. *Endoscopy* **19**(2): 64–67

Fisher ER, Sass R, Palekar A, Fisher B, Wolmark N (1989). Dukes' classification revisited. Findings from the National Surgical Adjuvant Breast and Bowel Projects (Protocol R-01). *Cancer* **64**, 2354–2360

Frykholm GJ, Pahlman L, Glimelius B (1995). Treatment of local recurrences of rectal carcinoma. *Radiotherapy & Oncology* **34**, 185–194

Garcia-Aguilar J, Mellgren A, Sirivongs P, Buie D, Madoff RD, Rothenberger DA (2000). Local excision of rectal cancer without adjuvant therapy: a word of caution. *Annals of Surgery* **231**, 345–351

Goldstein NS & Hart J (1999). Histologic features associated with lymph node metastasis in stage T1 and superficial T2 rectal adenocarcinomas in abdominoperineal resection specimens. Identifying a subset of patients for whom treatment with adjuvant therapy or completion abdominoperineal resection should be considered after local excision. *American Journal of Clinical Pathology* **111**, 51–58

Grinnell RS (1939). The grading and prognosis of carcinoma of the colon and rectum. *Annals of Surgery* **109**, 500–533

Gualdi GF, Casciani E, Guadalaxara A, d'Orta C, Polettini E, Pappalardo G (2000). Local staging of rectal cancer with transrectal ultrasound and endorectal magnetic resonance imaging: comparison with histologic findings. *Diseases of the Colon & Rectum* **43**, 338–345

Harrison JC, Dean PJ, el-Zeky F, Vander Zwaag R (1994). From Dukes through Jass: pathological prognostic indicators in rectal cancer [see comments]. *Human Pathology* **25**, 498–505

Heald RJ (1995). Total mesorectal excision is optimal surgery for rectal cancer: a Scandinavian consensus *British Journal of Surgery* **82**, 1297–1299

Heald RJ, Moran BJ, Ryall RD, Sexton R, MacFarlane JK (1998). Rectal cancer: the Basingstoke experience of total mesorectal excision, 1978–1997. *Archives of Surgery* **133**, 894–899

Hermanek P, Henson DE, Hutter RVP, Sobin LH (eds) (1993). *UICC TNM supplement 1993. A commentary on uniform use.* Berlin: Springer

Holm T, Johansson H, Cedermark B, Ekelund G, Rutqvist LE (1997). Influence of hospital- and surgeon-related factors on outcome after treatment of rectal cancer with or without preoperative radiotherapy. *British Journal of Surgery* **84**, 657–663

Horn A, Dahl O, Morild I (1990). The role of venous and neural invasion on survival in rectal adenocarcinoma. *Diseases of the Colon & Rectum* **33**, 598–601

Horn A, Dahl O, Morild I (1991). Venous and neural invasion as predictors of recurrence in rectal adenocarcinoma. *Diseases of the Colon & Rectum* **34**, 798–804

Hughes TG, Jenevein EP, Poulos E (1983). Intramural spread of colon carcinoma. A pathologic study. *American Journal of Surgery* **146**, 697–699

Hulsmans FJH, Tio TL, Fockens P, Bosma A, Tytgat GNJ (1994). Assessment of tumor infiltration depth in rectal cancer with transrectal sonography: caution is necessary. *Radiology* **190**, 715–720

Jass JR (1986). Lymphocytic infiltration and survival in rectal cancer. *Journal of Clinical Pathology* **39**, 585–589

Jass JR & Love SB (1989). Prognostic value of direct spread in Dukes' C cases of rectal cancer. *Diseases of the Colon & Rectum* **32**, 477–480

Jass JR, Atkin WS, Cuzick J *et al.* (1986). The grading of rectal cancer: historical perspectives and a multivariate analysis of 447 cases. *Histopathology* **10**, 437–459

Katsura Y, Yamada K, Ishizawa T, Yoshinaka H, Shimazu H (1992). Endorectal ultrasonography for the assessment of wall invasion and lymph node metastases in rectal cancer. *Diseases of the Colon & Rectum* **35**, 362–368

Kim NK, Kim MJ, Yun SH, Sohn SK, Min JS (1999). Comparative study of transrectal ultrasonography, pelvic computerized tomography, and magnetic resonance imaging in preoperative staging of rectal cancer. *Diseases of the Colon & Rectum* **42**, 770–775

Kusunoki M, Yanagi H, Kamikonya N *et al*. (1994). Preoperative detection of local extension of carcinoma of the rectum using magnetic resonance imaging. *Journal of the American College of Surgeons* **179**, 653–656

Lindmark G, Elvin A, Pahlman L, Glimelius B (1992). The value of endosonography in preoperative staging of rectal cancer. *International Journal of Colorectal Disease* **7**, 162–166

Lindmark G, Gerdin B, Pahlman L, Bergstrom R, Glimelius B (1994). Prognostic Predictors In Colorectal Cancer. *Diseases of the Colon & Rectum* **37**, 1219–1277

McNicholas MM, Joyce WP, Dolan J, Gibney RG, MacErlaine DP, Hyland J (1994). Magnetic resonance imaging of rectal carcinoma: a prospective study. *British Journal of Surgery* **81**, 911–914

Madsen PM & Christiansen J (1986). Distal intramural spread of rectal carcinomas. *Diseases of the Colon & Rectum* **29**, 279–282

Maldjian C, Smith R, Kilger A, Schnall M, Ginsberg G, Kochman M (2000). Endorectal surface coil MR imaging as a staging technique for rectal carcinoma: a comparison study to rectal endosonography. *Abdominal Imaging* **25**, 75–80

Marsh PJ, James RD, Schofield PF (1994). Adjuvant preoperative radiotherapy for locally advanced rectal carcinoma. results of a prospective, randomized trial. *Disease of the Colon & Rectum* **37**, 1205–1214

Mehta S, Johnson RJ, Schofield PF (1994). Staging of colorectal cancer. *Clinical Radiology* **49**, 515–523

Moran MR, James EC, Rothenberger DA, Goldberg SM (1992). Prognostic value of positive lymph nodes in rectal cancer. *Diseases of the Colon & Rectum* **35**, 579–581

Neymark N & Adriaenssen I (1999). The cost of managing patients with advanced colorectal cancer in 10 different European centres. *European Journal of Cancer* **35**, 1789–1795

Pahlman L (1998). Radiochemotherapy as an adjuvant treatment for rectal cancer. *Recent Results in Cancer Research* **146**, 141–151

Quirke P & Dixon MF (1988). The prediction of local recurrence in rectal adenocarcinoma by histopathological examination. *International Journal of Colorectal Disease* **3**, 127–131

Quirke P, Durdey P, Dixon MF, Williams NS (1986). Local recurrence of rectal adenocarcinoma due to inadequate surgical resection. Histopathological study of lateral tumour spread and surgical excision. *The Lancet* **ii**, 996–999

Rich T, Gunderson LL, Lew R, Galdibini JJ, Cohen AM, Donaldson G (1983). Patterns of recurrence of rectal cancer after potentially curative surgery. *Cancer* **52**, 1317–1329

Rifkin MD & Marks GJ (1985). Transrectal US as an adjunct in the diagnosis of rectal and extrarectal tumors. *Radiology* **157**, 499–502

Royal College of Surgeons and the Association of Coloproctology of Great Britain and Ireland (1996). *Guidelines for the Management of Colorectal Cancer*. Royal College Of Surgeons and the Association of Coloproctology of Great Britain and Ireland

Schnall MD, Furth EE, Rosato EF, Kressel HY (1994). Rectal tumor stage: correlation of endorectal MR imaging and pathologic findings *Radiology* **190**, 709–714

Shepherd NA, Baxter KJ, Love SB (1995). Influence of local peritoneal involvement on pelvic recurrence and prognosis in rectal cancer. *Journal of Clinical Pathology* **48**, 849–855

Sidoni A, Bufalari A, Alberti PF (1991). Distal intramural spread in colorectal cancer: a reappraisal of the extent of distal clearance in fifty cases. *Tumori* **77**, 514–517

Sobin LH & Wittekind C (eds) (1997). *TNM Classification of Malignant Tumours*, 5th edn. New York: John Wiley & Sons, Inc., p 227

Spinelli P, Schiavo M *et al*. (1999). Results of EUS in detecting perirectal lymph node metastases of rectal cancer: the pathologist makes the difference. *Gastrointestinal Endoscopy* **49**, 754–758

Spratt JA & Spjut HJ (1967). Prevalence and prognosis of carcinoma of the colon and rectum. *Cancer* **20**, 1976–1985

Swedish Rectal Cancer Trial (1997). Improved survival with preoperative radiotherapy in resectable rectal cancer. *New England Journal of Medicine* **336**, 980–987

Talbot IC, Ritchie S, Leighton M, Hughes AO, Bussey HJR, Morson BC (1981). Invasion of veins by carcinoma of rectum: method of detection, histological features and significance. *Histopathology* **5**, 141

Urban M, Rosen HR, Holbling N *et al*. (2000). MR imaging for the preoperative planning of sphincter-saving surgery for tumors of the lower third of the rectum: use of intravenous and endorectal contrast materials. *Radiology* **214**, 503–508

Wallengren NO, Holtas S, Andren-Sandberg A, Jonsson E, Kristoffersson DT, McGill S (2000). Rectal carcinoma: double-contrast MR imaging for preoperative staging. *Radiology* **215**, 108–114

Wolmark N, Fisher ER, Wieand HS, Fisher B (1984). The relationship of depth of penetration and tumor size to the number of positive nodes in Dukes C colorectal cancer. *Cancer* **53**, 2707–2712

Zerhouni EA, Rutter C, Hamilton SR *et al*. (1996). T and MR imaging in the staging of colorectal carcinoma: report of the Radiology Diagnostic Oncology Group II. *Radiology* **200**, 443–451

Chapter 11

Current thinking on the utility of preoperative chemoradiation

David Sebag-Montefiore

Introduction

There is increasing use of preoperative radiotherapy in Europe. The reasons for this include the aim of reducing local recurrence, increasing the proportion of sphincter-preserving resections and possibly improving survival. As there is more than one aim, it is perhaps not surprising that there is confusion surrounding the specific role of preoperative concurrent chemoradiotherapy (CRT). There are specific problems that relate to preoperative staging, the choice of radiotherapy schedule and the optimal chemoradiotherapy regimen.

Preoperative local staging of rectal cancer

The local extent of a rectal carcinoma can range from a small focus of malignancy arising within an adenoma to a large fixed tumour that has breached the mesorectal fascia to invade surrounding structures directly. Local disease extent can be assessed by digital rectal examination (DRE), transrectal ultrasonography (TRUS) or cross-sectional imaging using either computed tomography (CT) or magnetic resonance imaging (MRI).

The first MRC adjuvant radiotherapy trial (Anonymous 1984) demonstrated that clinicians using DRE could identify patients with fixed tumours who had a worse prognosis. Nichols *et al.* (1982) evaluated the role of DRE in a single institution and concluded that the 'educated finger' of an experienced coloproctologist could identify patients with locally advanced disease. However, DRE has limitations, including the inability to assess tumours in the upper half of the rectum, which is beyond the length of the examining finger, and the subjective nature of the assessment.

Transrectal ultrasonography has been accepted as the imaging 'gold standard' for the assessment of the local tumour (T) stage, but again has limitations in the assessment of more advanced disease, e.g. the tumour may be circumferential and stenosing, precluding the passage of the ultrasonic probe through the lesion, or the patient may not be able to tolerate the procedure. The field of view is also limited, precluding useful assessment of long bulky tumours, and it is operator dependent.

Recently there has been particular interest in the role of MRI. This has developed in parallel with the improvements on the surgical techniques employed in the resection of rectal cancer. The use of sharp dissection, including total mesorectal excision

(TME) as described by Heald (MacFarlane *et al.* 1993), and the simple yet elegant methods of histopathological examination of the resected specimen, described by Quirke (Adam *et al.* 1994), represent major advances. It has increased our understanding of both the mechanism of local recurrence and how its incidence might be reduced by improved surgical technique. This has focused clinicians on the importance of the relationship of the tumour to the lateral (circumferential) resection margin.

The mesorectum, primary tumour and lymph nodes are all demonstrated on high-quality pelvic MR images when performed under the supervision of specialist radiologists. It is also possible to identify the mesorectal envelope, and for the first time reliably demonstrate the anatomical 'package' that should be removed by TME (Figure 11.1).

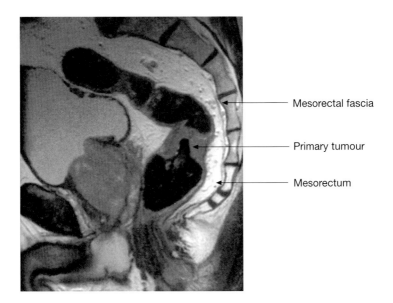

Mesorectal fascia

Primary tumour

Mesorectum

Figure 11.1 Sagittal MRI scan demonstrating a rectal carcinoma, the surrounding mesorectal fat and the mesorectal fascia representing the intended plane of surgical excision when a mesorectal excision is performed.

A number of studies have recently evaluated the role of MRI in the preoperative assessment of rectal cancer (Brown *et al.* 1999; Beets-Tan *et al.* 2001; Bissett *et al.* 2001; Botterill *et al.* 2001). Brown *et al.* (1999), in an elegant prospective study, compared preoperative MRI findings with ultra-thin whole histopathology mounts using the techniques of Quirke in 28 patients. This study clearly demonstrated the mesorectal fascia and the relationship of the tumour to it. There was a high degree of correlation in T stage and measurements of the depth of extramural tumour extension.

Bissett *et al.* (2001) has provided further confirmation that the surgical fascia propria and any tumour extension beyond it can be reliably identified on MRI. In a retrospective study from Leeds by Botterill *et al.* (2001), the use of MRI in a multidisciplinary setting provided further information on the probability of circumferential resection margin (CRM) involvement; 61 patients proceeded to initial surgery, of whom only 5 (8%) were found to have histopathological involvement of the CRM.

In a recent retrospective study from the Netherlands, Beets-Tan *et al.* (2001) used MRI to predict CRM involvement and divided patients into three groups:

1. Predicted margin involvement.
2. Predicted clear margin by > 10 mm.
3. An intermediate group.

The regression analysis of the intermediate group suggested that 5-mm clearance of tumour from the predicted CRM on MRI needed to achieve a greater than 95% probability of more than 1-mm clearance of the histopathological CRM. Further studies are required to demonstrate the accuracy of MRI in defining preoperatively the primary T stage and the distance of tumour to the intended circumferential resection margin (the mesorectal fascia).

Prospective studies are also required to evaluate its role as a method of patient selection for preoperative radiotherapy. Should these studies prove successful, then for the first time an objective imaging classification could be used to stratify patients by disease extent, including the proximity to the mesorectal fascia.

Short- or long-course radiotherapy?

The results of the Swedish Rectal Cancer trial (Anonymous 1997) have clearly influenced clinical practice for patients with resectable rectal cancer. This trial demonstrated a statistically significant improvement in overall survival, as well as a reduction in local recurrence. However, there have been significant improvements in surgical technique and histopathological examination of the resected specimen requiring further trials to examine the role of short-course preoperative radiotherapy in resectable rectal cancer. The Dutch TME trial and the MRC CR07 trials both compare a policy of routine short-course radiotherapy with initial surgery to that of initial TME and selective postoperative radiotherapy for patients with an involved CRM.

The Dutch trial (Kapiteijn *et al.* 2001) recruited more than 1,800 patients and the MRC CR07 trial, which is continuing to recruit, has randomised over 600 patients. The two trials have very similar rates of circumferential margin involvement, anastomotic leak, abdominoperineal excision and the histopathological assessment of the quality of surgery (Kapiteijn *et al.* 1999; Sebag-Montefiore 2001).

These very important trials will establish the size of any benefit when using routine short-course preoperative radiotherapy in combination with modern surgical and histopathological techniques.

The Dutch trial has recently been published and reports a reduction in actuarial 2-year local recurrence rate from 8.2% with initial TME to 2.4% with the addition of short-course preoperative radiotherapy (SCPRT) (Kapiteijn *et al*. 2001). The median follow-up is relatively short at 25 months and it is too early to consider overall survival. Intriguingly, there are some clues in hypothesis-generating subset analysis where short-course preoperative radiotherapy is less effective. An important caveat is that any subgroup analysis requires confirmation from prospective studies such as the CR07 trial. SCPRT did not significantly reduce the risk of local recurrence in the minority of patients with an involved CRM when compared with initial TME (approximately half of these patients received postoperative radiotherapy). This may be a group of patients for whom MRI may be able to predict recurrence and who could be considered for preoperative chemoradiotherapy studies.

Postoperative radiotherapy or chemoradiotherapy?

There is still controversy surrounding the perceived benefit of concurrent CRT when compared with radiotherapy alone. This is mainly the result of the lack of randomised controlled trials addressing this specific question. Most trials have been performed in the postoperative setting in North America.

In resectable rectal cancer, Krook *et al*. (1991) randomised 204 patients after resection of T3/4 or node-positive rectal cancer to receive either concurrent (and sequential) chemotherapy in combination with radiotherapy or radiotherapy alone, and demonstrated a highly statistically significant reduction in local recurrence and improved survival. A difficulty in interpreting this study is that the addition of sequential and concurrent chemotherapy to radiotherapy was compared with radiotherapy alone, and thus prevents assessment of the relative contribution of the sequential and concurrent chemotherapy components.

The subsequent study used sequential and concurrent chemotherapy in combination with radiotherapy in both arms (O'Connell *et al*. 1994). In this study the comparison was between bolus 5-fluorouracil (5FU) and continuous infusion 5FU during radiotherapy (PVI-5FU). Local recurrence was low in both arms, but there was a statistically significant improvement in survival in favour of PVI-5FU. One way of interpreting the survival advantage seen in this study is that the delivery of PVI-5FU allowed more dose-intense and effective chemotherapy to continue during radiotherapy.

The National Surgical Adjuvant Breast and Bowel Project (NSABP) R02 study (Woolmark *et al*. 2000) was complex in design as a result of the need to use different chemotherapy control arms for men and women, based on the results of the previous R01 trial. Despite this, there was a randomised comparison between chemotherapy alone and chemotherapy + concurrent chemoradiotherapy (C + CRT) (unlike the

Krook study where the control arm consisted of radiotherapy alone). This study demonstrated a statistically significant reduction in local recurrence (as first event) of 13% compared with 8% in favour of the C + CRT arm, but no difference in overall survival.

It is worth reading the report of this trial carefully. It is clear that, similar to the Krook study, the concurrent chemotherapy consisted of bolus 5FU during 3 days of the first and fifth weeks of radiotherapy. There was also a gap after completion of CRT before systemic chemotherapy recommenced. These interruptions in 5FU dose intensity will not have occurred in the CT-alone arm.

When these three trials are considered together, there is some evidence to suggest that delivering relatively more intensive 5FU during radiotherapy may influence survival. One of the key reasons that doubt remains as to whether systemic chemotherapy alone improves survival in rectal cancer may be a result of the uncontrolled use of adjuvant radiotherapy. Major interruptions in useful systemic chemotherapy delivery occur either because of a lower dose and dose intensity of chemotherapy during CRT and the interruptions in systemic chemotherapy delivery both before and after radiotherapy.

Preoperative radiotherapy or chemoradiotherapy?

There have been very few randomised controlled trials that have compared preoperative radiotherapy alone with concurrent chemoradiotherapy. One very small study in patients with fixed non-resectable rectal cancer has recently been published and, as a result of the rarity of such a trial, deserves discussion (Frykholm *et al.* 2001); 70 patients were recruited over 8 years and randomised to receive either 46 Gy in 23 fractions (RT alone) or concurrent chemoradiotherapy (40 Gy + methotrexate, 5FU and leucovorin [LV]). The CRT regimen was based on previous pilot data and it should be noted that this study commenced in 1988. However, the CRT regimen would be considered suboptimal today for many reasons, e.g. radiotherapy was given as 10 Gy in five fractions over 3 days and repeated alternate weeks, with an overall treatment time of 45 days.

Despite the deficiencies in the CRT schedule, there was a higher rate of resection and a statistically significant lower rate of local recurrence in favour of the CRT arm (for curative resections and all patients who underwent resection). Overall local control was improved with the use of CRT when all patients were included in the analysis. Despite its limitations, this is an important small trial that demonstrates a benefit for CRT when compared with radiotherapy alone in fixed inoperable rectal cancer.

The European Organization for Research and Treatment of Cancer (EORTC) is conducting a trial (22921) comparing preoperative radiotherapy (45 Gy) with preoperative CRT in patients with resectable rectal cancer, with a second randomisation evaluating the benefit of the addition of four cycles of 5FU–LV compared with no further treatment. It is hoped that 1,000 patients will be recruited. This trial is likely to help answer the benefit of CRT over RT alone in resectable disease.

End-points: what should be measured?

Many phase II studies of CRT are published every year. Interpretation of these data is difficult as a result of the problems already alluded to in the objective measurement of the extent of disease. However, most studies report acute toxicity and histopathological stage, and relatively few have any information on local recurrence or survival.

Many clinicians focus on the rate of pathological complete response (pCR), considering this to be the most important surrogate measure of outcome. It is, of course, essential that the highest pCR rate is obtained if the aim is to move from a preoperative combined modality approach to that of definitive chemoradiation alone. It is clear that, although this has been achieved in the management of anal cancer, this step will require major improvements of the chemoradiation schedule before it is even considered in rectal cancer.

When CRT is given preoperatively in locally advanced rectal cancer, the main aims are to facilitate macroscopic tumour shrinkage to allow resection and minimise the risk of local recurrence. A further aim might include the treatment of microscopic metastatic disease beyond the pelvis, but it is important to note that current CRT schedules commonly restrict chemotherapy delivery to the 5 weeks of radiation and also use suboptimal doses of chemotherapy (when compared with that used as systemic treatment alone). The improvement of CRT schedules to address this deficiency should be the subject of future clinical trials.

If one considers the issues of achieving resection and minimising local recurrence with the current CRT regimens, what surrogate end-points are most important? First, it is important that published results describe all patients treated, because a proportion will remain irresectable after CRT. Second, those patients who undergo resection may be classified as R2 (macroscopic residual disease), R1 (microscopic residual disease) and R0 (histologically confirmed clear margins). The concept of the R0 resection has been refined further by the techniques of Quirke where a R0 resection using this technique requires that the CRM is uninvolved. This is defined as microscopic tumour that is not within 1 mm of the CRM.

Current CRT published reports rarely identify all these individual steps in the analysis. It is also common for an R0 resection to be based only on clear proximal and distal resection margins, because the histopathological techniques of Quirke have not been used. The recent data from the Dutch trial in resectable disease show that, with the use of TME and Quirke's techniques, only 77% of patients were found to have tumour-free margins.

All these factors can be included in the assessment of a CRT regimen, and the experience from the Leeds Cancer Network (Cooper & Sebag-Montefiore 2000) is used to illustrate these features (Figure 11.2). A total of 63 patients with locally advanced rectal cancer received CRT using 5FU and folinic acid, described by Bosset *et al.* (1993). Ten patients were considered irresectable after CRT, and nine underwent a R2 resection, leaving a total of 44 patients who underwent a potentially curative resection in the opinion of the surgeon (of whom 25% were found to have involvement of the CRM) (Figure 11.2).

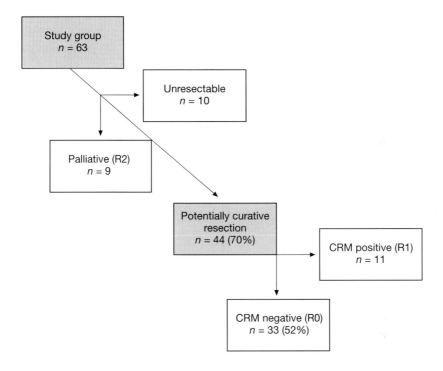

Figure 11.2 Flow diagram of patients treated by CRT with locally advanced rectal cancer demonstrating that 52% of the whole group underwent a histologically confirmed curative (R0) resection.

The measures of efficacy for this group of patients is shown in Table 11.1. It is interesting that, with a relatively short median follow-up of 25 months, no local recurrences have been detected in the patients who underwent a R0 resection with histological confirmation of an uninvolved CRM (CRM-negative R0). In this series 52% of the original study group underwent a CRM-negative R0 resection. It would be most interesting to analyse future CRT studies using a method similar to that shown in Figure 11.2. Despite the large numbers of published studies of CRT, there is a disappointingly small number that report local recurrence and survival. There are important, and as yet unanswered, questions relating to the outcome of patients, e.g. it would be helpful if the larger studies reported outcome stratified by histopathological stage (pCR, pT1N0 and pT1/2N0 disease).

Table 11.1 Measures of efficacy of preoperative chemoradiotherapy using the Bosset regimen with Leeds Cancer Network data

Histopathological complete response	15%
pT0/2N0	32%
R0 resection (patients who underwent potentially curative resection)	75%
Local recurrence (patients who underwent potentially curative resection)	9%
R0 resection (whole study group)	53%

The author wishes to highlight that investigators of novel chemoradiation regimens will need to derive, if possible, early surrogate end-points to help to compare the multitude of different options for selecting the regimens to be tested in future phase III trials. It is not clear at present whether this should be based on the rate of 'downstaging' – pCR, pT0/1N0 or pT0/2N0. It is also unclear what the prognostic implications are when a major treatment effect is seen, but the minor residual foci of cancer do not alter the pre-treatment stage, e.g. if a patient with T3 disease on TRUS received preoperative CRT and the histopathological specimen shows that a few foci remained in perirectal fat, this would still represent pT3 disease even though over 99% of all tumour had disappeared within 6 weeks. Does this group of patients have a lower risk of recurrence compared with those in whom there is no evidence of a treatment effect? The data from Janjan *et al.* (1999) support the view that the lack of T-stage 'downstaging' is associated with a poorer outcome.

An alternative approach to assess the efficacy of a CRT regimen is the proportion of patients with a clear CRM (CRM-negative R0). This would be most convincing in conjunction with preoperative MRI prediction of the proximity of the tumour to the CRM.

Novel chemoradiation regimens

This section aims to provide an overview of recent reports of new regimens. This is not an inclusive review and attempts to highlight the direction of this area of research. Many of these reports are currently in abstract form, and should be regarded as preliminary reports with the publication of the data awaited in a peer-reviewed journal. Although standard CRT is based on the combination of intravenous 5FU with radiation, a number of alternative single-agent approaches have recently been reported.

Single-agent studies

Oral fluoropyrimidines

The oral fluoropyrimidines offer the major convenience of oral therapy, and their use overcomes many of the difficulties of delivering 5FU intravenously with radiation. The logistic difficulties of delivering 5FU-based CRT should not be underestimated. The use of PVI-5FU requires the inconvenience of infusion pumps and the associated risks of indwelling lines for central drug delivery. Alternatively, the use of short infusion or bolus 5FU requires close scheduling with the delivery of radiation, with its attendant problems.

The oral fluoropyrimidines capecitabine (Dunst & Frings 2001; Ngan *et al.* 2001), oral uracil and tegafur (UFT) (Pfeiffer 2000; Fernandez-Martos *et al.* 2001) and eniluracil (Cohen *et al.* 2000) have all been combined with radiation in phase I studies. The study by Dunst and Frings has used a continuous schedule of capecitabine given orally twice daily over 5 weeks and found the maximum tolerated dose (MTD) of capecitabine to be 1,000 mg/m^2 twice daily every day, when combined with 45-Gy radiotherapy plus a 5.4-Gy boost. The dose-limiting toxicity is hand–foot syndrome and the recommended dose for phase II studies is 825 mg/m^2 twice daily. The study by Ngan *et al.* used twice daily capecitabine only during the 5 days of radiation and has not yet reached dose-limiting toxicity (DLT) at 1,000 mg/m^2 twice daily orally and, at the time of writing, continues to recruit.

Pfeiffer (2000) reported a phase I/II study that gave 60 Gy of irradiation with a 5 days/week dose-escalating schedule of UFT (150–300 mg/m^2 per day) with a fixed dose of isovorin 7.5 mg and recently Fernandez-Martos *et al.* (2001) have reported a phase II study using UFT 400 mg/m^2 5 days per week with 45 Gy of radiation preoperatively.

A phase I study that dose escalated oral eniluracil/5FU twice daily using a continuous schedule with 45 Gy of radiation recommended 8 mg/m^2 to 0.8 mg/m^2 as a recommended dose for phase II studies.

Other single-agent studies

Two phase I studies of CRT using single-agent raltitrexed have been reported. Valentini *et al.* (1999) reported that the MTD had not been reached when raltitrexed was given at 3 mg/m^2 on days 1, 19 and 37 with 50.4 Gy of irradiation. Similarly, James *et al.* (1999) dose escalated raltitrexed to 3 mg/m^2 given days 1 and 22 with 50 Gy of radiation.

Minsky *et al.* (1999) reported his experience of daily intravenous irinotecan with 50.4 Gy of radiation in locally advanced disease. The dose-limiting toxicity was diarrhoea and was experienced at 13 mg/m^2 per day; the MTD was established as 10 mg/m^2 per day.

It seems unlikely that further studies of either single-agent raltitrexed or irinotecan combined with radiation will be of great benefit. More interest surrounds the development of combination chemotherapy schedules, building on their success in metastatic disease and their integration with radiation.

Combination schedules

The majority of combination schedules consist of a phase I study where a second drug (irinotecan, oxaliplatin or mitomycin C) is dose escalated with a fixed dose of 5FU and radiation. Two European studies have reported the combination of oxaliplatin with 5FU and radiation. The Lyon study (Freyer 2001) which has been recently published and the Colorectal Clinical Oncology Group (CCOG) study (Sebag-Montefiore *et al.* 2001) in abstract form have recommended the dose of oxaliplatin for phase II combination studies as 130 mg/m^2 when given during the first and fifth weeks of radiation. The CCOG study added oxaliplatin to the established 5FU/FA (folinic acid) regimen described by Bosset *et al.* (1993), with 45 Gy of irradiation – which is the novel CRT arm of the current EORTC trial described above. In contrast, the Lyon regimen uses a 24-hour infusion of 5FU in combination with FA on days 1–5 and 29–33 and increased the radiation dose to 50.4 Gy. The dose-limiting toxicities in the CCOG study consisted of diarrhoea and neurotoxiciy.

Valentini *et al.* (2001) have recently reported in abstract form a phase I study in which the dose of oxaliplatin was dose escalated on days 1, 19 and 38, with a fixed dose of raltitrexed 3 mg/m^2 and 50.4 Gy of radiation. This study has also recommended the dose of oxaliplatin as 130 mg/m^2 for phase II combination studies with this regimen.

A number of phase I studies have also been performed where the dose of irinotecan has been escalated with a fixed dose of 5FU and radiation. Mitchell *et al.* (2001) have updated their experience in abstract form, where irinotecan was given on days 1, 8, 15 and 22 in combination with PVI–5FU and radiation. It proved necessary to de-escalate the dose of PVI–5FU to allow full-dose escalation of irinotecan. The MTD of irinotecan is 50 mg/m^2 when combined with 54 Gy of radiation and 225 mg/m^2 5FU given 5 days/week. The dose-limiting toxicities were diarrhoea and intravenous catheter-related complications. Mehta *et al.* (2001) have reported a small phase II study using a similar regimen, but with a lower dose of PVI–5FU (200 mg/m^2 per day) and lower dose of radiation (45–50.4 Gy).

The CCOG is studying the dose escalation of irinotecan on days 1–5 and 29–33 when added to the Bosset regimen, and a phase I study where the dose of mitomycin C is dose escalated when added to PVI–5FU and 45 Gy of irradiation.

Further studies are under way in many countries, establishing the regimens for phase II trials, and many phase II studies will commence in 2002. These studies will have a number of variations, including significant differences in the dose intensity and dose of the novel drug that has been integrated into the CRT regimen and the dose of radiation. There will also be studies where the combination schedule uses an oral fluoropyrimidine to replace intravenous 5FU, again with different delivery schedules.

Conclusion

There is considerable promise that MRI scanning will allow the development of a preoperative objective staging system for rectal cancer and influence the decision-making process of selecting patients for preoperative radiotherapy.

The results of the published Dutch TME trial and the ongoing MRC CR07 and EORTC 22921 studies will influence the future use of preoperative CRT.

The rapid increase in the number of phase I and phase II chemoradiation studies will be followed by the need to solve the problem of deriving early surrogate endpoints, to allow randomised phase II studies to determine the best regimens to take forward into future phase III trials.

References

Adam IJ, Mohamdee MO, Martin IG *et al*. (1994). Role of circumferential margin involvement in the local recurrence of rectal cancer. *The Lancet* **344**, 707–711

Anonymous (1984). The evaluation of low dose pre-operative X ray therapy in the management of operable rectal cancer; results of a randomly controlled trial. *British Journal of Surgery* **71**, 21–25

Anonymous (1997). Improved survival with preoperative radiotherapy in resectable rectal cancer. *New England Journal of Medicine* **336**, 980–987

Beets-Tan RGH, Beets GL, Vliegen RFA *et al*. (2001). Accuracy of magnetic resonance imaging in prediction of tumour-free resection margin in rectal cancer surgery. *The Lancet* **357**, 497–504

Bissett IP, Fernando CC, Hough DM *et al*. (2001). Identification of the fascia propria by magnetic resonance imaging and its relevance to pre operative assessment of rectal cancer. *Diseases of Colon and Rectum* **44**, 259–265

Bosset JF, Pavy JJ, Hamers HP *et al*. (1993). Determination of the optimal dose of 5 fluorouracil when combined with low dose D,L-leucovorin and irradiation in rectal cancer: results of three consecutive phase II studies. *European Journal of Cancer* **29A**, 1406–1410

Botterill ID, Blunt DM, Quirke P *et al*. (2001). Evaluation of the role of pre-operative magnetic resonance imaging in the management of rectal cancer. *International Journal of Colorectal Disease* **3**, 295–304

Brown G, Richards CJ, Newcombe RG *et al*. (1999). Rectal carcinoma: thin-section MR imaging for staging in 28 patients. *Radiology* **211**, 215–222

Cohen DP, Lee CG, Anscher MS *et al*. (2000). Phase I study of chemoradiation therapy with oral eniluracil (776C85)/5 Fluorouracil in patients with rectal adenocarcinoma. *Proceedings of the American Society of Clinical Oncology*, Abstract 1013

Cooper R & Sebag-Montefiore D (2000). Pre-operative chemoradiotherapy for locally advanced carcinoma of the rectum: acute toxicity, pathological response and outcome. *Radiotherapy and Oncology* **56**(S1): 257

Dunst J & Frings S (2001). Phase I study of Capecitabine combined with simultaneous radiotherapy in rectal cancer. *Proceedings of the American Society of Clinical Oncology*, Abstract 591

Fernandez-Martos C, Aparicio J, Bosch C *et al*. (2001). Pre-operative therapy with oral uracil and tegafur (UFT) and concomitant irradiation in operable rectal cancer. Preliminary results of a multicentre phase II study. *Proceedings of the American Society of Clinical Oncology*, Abstract 590.

Freyer G, Bossard N, Thornestaing P *et al*. (2001). Addition of oxaliplatin to continuous fluorouracil, L-folinic acid and concomitant radiotherapy in rectal cancer: The Lyon R97-03 phase I trial. *Journal of Clinical Oncology* **19**, 2433–2438

Frykholm GJ, Pahlman L, Glimelius B (2001). Combined chemo and radiotherapy vs radiotherapy alone in the treatment of primary, non resectable adenocarcinoma of the rectum. *International Journal of Radiation Oncology Biology Physics* **50**, 433–440

James RD, Price P, Smith M (1999). Raltitrexed (Tomudex) plus radiotherapy is well tolerated and warrants further investigation in patients with advanced inoperable/ recurrent rectal cancer. *Proceedings of the American Society of Clinical Oncology*, Abstract 1105

Janjan NA, Abbruzzese J, Pazdur R *et al*. (1999). Prognostic implications of response to preoperative infusional chemoradiation in locally advanced rectal cancer. *Radiotherapy and Oncology* **51**, 153–160

Kapiteijn E, Kranenbarg EK, Steup WH *et al*. (1999). Total mesorectal excision (TME) with or without preoperative radiotherapy in the treatment of primary rectal cancer: prospective randomised trial with standard operative and histopathological techniques *European Journal of Surgery* **165**, 410–420

Kapiteijn E, Marijnen CAM, Nagtegaal ID *et al*. (2001). Preoperative radiotherapy combined with total mesorectal excision for resectable rectal cancer. *New England Journal of Medicine* **345**, 638–646

Krook JE, Moertel CG, Gunderson LL *et al*. (1991). Effective surgical adjuvant therapy for high risk rectal carcinoma. *New England Journal of Medicine* **324**, 709–715

MacFarlane JK, Ryall RDH, Heald RJ (1993). Mesorectal excision for rectal cancer. *The Lancet* **341**, 457–460

Mehta VK, Fisher G, Cho C *et al*. (2001). Phase II trial of preoperative radiotherapy, protracted venous infusion 5FU and weekly CPT-11, followed by surgery for ultrasound staged T3/T4 rectal cancer. *Proceedings of the American Society of Clinical Oncology*, Abstract 590.

Minsky BD, O'Reilly E, Wong D *et al*. (1999). Daily low dose irinotecan (CPT-11) plus pelvic irradiation as preoperative treatment of locally advanced rectal cancer. *Proceedings of the American Society of Clinical Oncology*, Abstract 1023

Mitchell EP, Anne P, Fry R *et al*. (2001). Combined modality therapy of locally advanced or recurrent adenocarcinoma of the rectum: report of a phase I trial of chemotherapy with CPT11, 5FU and concomitant irradiation. *Proceedings of the American Society of Clinical Oncology*, Abstract 519

Ngan S, Zalcberg J, Kell A *et al*. (2001). A phase I study of Capecitabine combined with radiotherapy for locally advanced potentially operable rectal cancer. *Proceedings of the American Society of Clinical Oncology*, Abstract 591

Nicholls RJ, York Mason A, Morson BC, Dixon AK, Kelsey Fry I (1982). The clinical staging of rectal cancer *British Journal of Surgery* **69**, 404–409

O'Connell MJ, Martenson JA, Wieand HS *et al*. (1994). Improving adjuvant therapy for rectal cancer by combining protracted infusion fluorouracil with radiation after curative surgery. *New England Journal of Medicine* **331**, 502–507

Pfeiffer P (2000). Concurrent UFT/L-Leucovorin and curative intended radiotherapy (60Gy) in patients with locally advanced rectal cancer: A Phase I/II trial. *Proceedings of the American Society of Clinical Oncology*, Abstract 992

Sebag-Montefiore D (2001). An update report on the MRC CR07 trial. *British Journal of Cancer* **85**(S1), 28

Sebag-Montefiore D, Maughan T, Falk S *et al*. (2001). A phase I dose escalation study of oxaliplatin when given in combination with 5-fluorouracil, low dose folinic acid and synchronous pre-operative radiotherapy in locally advanced rectal cancer. *Proceedings of the American Society of Clinical Oncology*, Abstract 585

Valentini V, Morganti AG, Fiorentino G *et al*. (1999). Chemoradiation with raltitrexed (Tomudex) and concomitant preoperative radiotherapy has potential in the treatment of stage II/III resectable rectal cancer. *Proceedings of the American Society of Clinical Oncology*, Abstract 987

Valentini V, Morganti AG, Smaniotto D *et al.* (2001). Chemoradiation with raltitrexed (Tomudex) and oxaliplatin in pre-operative treatment of stage II/III resectable rectal cancer: a dose finding study. *Proceedings of the American Society of Clinical Oncology*, Abstract 520

Woolmark N, Wickerham DL, Fisher ER *et al.* (2000). Randomised trial of postoperative adjuvant chemotherapy with or without radiotherapy for carcinoma of the rectum: National Adjuvant Breast and Bowel Project Protocol R02. *Journal of the National Cancer Institute* **92**, 388–396

PART 4

NHS policy and colorectal cancer

Strategies for the efficient management of all patients with lower gastrointestinal symptoms to achieve effective diagnosis of colorectal cancer

Michael R Thompson, ET Swarbrick, BG Ellis, I Heath, L Faulds Wood, C Coles and WS Atkin

Introduction

It is usual and understandable to emphasise the importance of prompt and effective diagnosis of colorectal cancer when considering the management of patients presenting with lower gastrointestinal (GI) symptoms. However, because of the high prevalence of these symptoms in the community and primary care and the limited current resources for their investigation, this cannot be achieved without the efficient management of all these patients, with the majority who have transient symptoms not being referred to hospital.

The new Department of Health referral guidelines for bowel cancer were developed to improve both the effectiveness and efficiency of diagnosis of colorectal cancer and proposed new management strategies based on the following observations:

- The high prevalence of gastrointestinal symptoms in the community and in primary care, and the current shortage of hospital resources, establish the need for careful selection of patients for investigation.
- The current selection process is probably mainly based on 'treat, watch and wait' strategies which result in most patients with transient and intermittent symptoms avoiding investigation.
- There is little evidence that even substantial time lags after the onset of symptoms and before treatment affect survival from colorectal cancer.
- Estimates of the risk of symptomatic patients having bowel cancer can be determined on the basis of symptoms and signs elicited by a simple history and examination.

This chapter reviews the evidence for these observations, which support a policy of different management strategies according to cancer risk, with prompt referral to hospital of those patients with persistently higher-risk symptoms and no or slow referral for those with transient, intermittent or low-risk symptoms. It also outlines the methods that have been used to identify the higher-risk criteria for the 'two-week standard', review the implications for the service organisation in terms of the resources needed to cover the expected increase in referrals, and finally review methods of dissemination of the guidelines to GPs to increase their effectiveness.

The high prevalence of the three primary symptoms of colorectal cancer

The very high prevalence of all symptoms in the community regardless of their nature has been known for some time (Wadsworth *et al.* 1971; Hannay 1979; Pearse & Crocker 1985). This means that most people, most of the time, have one or more symptoms, which they either self-treat or which resolve spontaneously without a medical consultation.

This is also true for the three primary symptoms of bowel cancer

- change in bowel habit
- rectal bleeding
- abdominal pain

(Connell *et al.* 1965; Milne & Williamson 1972; Jones 1976; Drossman *et al.* 1982; Silman *et al.* 1983; Farrands & Hardcastle 1984; Donald *et al.* 1985; Dent *et al.* 1986; Sandler & Drossman 1987; Everhart *et al.* 1989; Kewenter *et al.* 1989; Sonnenberg & Koch 1989; Sandler 1990; Byles *et al.* 1992; Heaton *et al.* 1992a, 1992b; Jones & Lydeard 1992; Kay *et al.* 1992; Muris *et al.* 1993, 1995, 1996; Curless *et al.* 1994; Fijten *et al.* 1994; Crosland & Jones 1995; Talley & Jones 1998; Thompson *et al.* 2000); those patients at present investigated in hospital represent the 'tip of the iceberg' of all patients with these symptoms (Heaton *et al.* 1992b; Drossman *et al.* 1982; Dent *et al.* 1986; Sandler & Drossman 1987; Sandler 1990; Jones & Lydeard 1992; Crosland & Jones 1995; Talley & Jones 1998; Thompson *et al.* 2000). This selection process occurs mainly at the patient/GP interface and only secondarily at the GP/ hospital interface. These observations have serious implications for public awareness campaigns and GP referral guidelines. The aim of these is to improve the selection process so that the majority of cancer patients are referred reasonably promptly, and most patients without cancer are managed in the community and primary care.

How do patients and GPs decide whether to seek further advice?

It is likely that the current ways many patients decide to seek medical help and GPs decide whether to refer to hospital are based on 'treat, watch and wait' strategies, with the assumption that most benign conditions get better or at least have non-progressive or intermittent symptoms, whereas most with cancer have persistent, more worrying symptoms.

In general practice 'treat, watch and wait' strategies (Sackett *et al.* 1991) together with 'safety-netting' (Neighbour 1987) are used for the management of most common symptoms. They are an integral part of the diagnostic process, form part of good medical practice and are the keystone of the GPs' 'gate-keeper role'. It is crucial that new guidelines support GPs in this important role.

When does the risk of cancer outweigh the risk and disadvantage of investigation?

Most doctors are now accustomed to balancing the benefits of treatment with its risks (Muir Gray 1997a) and recognise the need for randomised controlled trials before introducing screening programmes for colorectal cancer. They are less familiar with balancing the risks of investigation with its benefits when deciding whether to refer symptomatic patients at low risk of cancer to hospital. If the benefits of earlier diagnosis are small in the few with cancer, this has to be weighed against the overall disadvantages and risks of investigating all patients with these symptoms. Some of the disadvantages of investigation are listed in Table 12.1.

All these negative factors must be taken into account when deciding whether to investigate a patient at low risk of cancer, and in determining the extent and safest mode of investigating the colon and rectum. In a health system that is short of resources, it is also important not to forget that unnecessary and inappropriate referral and investigation of patients at very low risk of cancer may block and delay the investigation of higher-risk patients, including most of those with cancer.

The safest and most efficient mode of investigation of patients with lower gastrointestinal symptoms is flexible sigmoidoscopy (Waye 1995; Dodds & Thompson 1997). In one study of over 8,000 patients in a surgical outpatient clinic, diagnosis of virtually all the significant large bowel pathology was achieved by flexible sigmoidoscopy (Dodds & Thompson 1997). The residual risk of cancer after a normal flexible sigmoidoscopy (Dodds & Thompson 1997) in patients with lower GI symptoms and no other significant diagnostic factors may be so small that immediate further investigation with a barium enema or colonoscopy is inappropriate and will do more 'harm than good'.

Will earlier diagnosis after the onset of symptoms reduce the overall mortality from colorectal cancer?

> The term 'early', used so often in discussions of cancer therapy is generally applied inappropriately. Although 'early' refers to a dimension in time, the usual evidence assessed in the designation of 'early' comes mainly from anatomy not chronometry.
>
> Feinstein (1966)

It is now well established from screening studies that the diagnosis of early stage disease in largely asymptomatic individuals significantly reduces the overall death

Table 12.1 Disadvantages of over-investigation

Unnecessary worry of investigation and fear of cancer (Marshall 1996; Stewart-Brown & Farmer 1997)

Labelling (Haynes *et al.* 1978; MacDonald *et al.* 1984)

Physical harm
- Colonoscopy 1:17,000 deaths (Williams 1986; Waye *et al.* 1996)
- Barium enema 1:57,000 deaths (Blakeborough *et al.* 1997)
- False positives/unnecessary operations
- False negatives/delayed diagnosis

Consuming scarce resources
- Resulting in delay in investigation of those with cancer
- Opportunity costs
- Patient and carer's costs
  - Time off work
  - Travel costs

Medicolegal costs

rate from colorectal cancer (Hardcastle *et al.* 1996; Kronborg *et al.* 1996; Mandel *et al.* 1999). However, this must not be confused with the common assumption that *diagnosis early* after the onset of symptoms will also result in the diagnosis of *earlier stage* disease with improved survival. Although this at first sight seems logical and there have been a few studies that have supported this idea (Welch & Burke 1962; Rowe-Jones & Aylett 1965; Rubin *et al.* 1980; MacArthur & Smith 1984; Robinson *et al.* 1986; Clarke *et al.* 1992; Launoy *et al.* 1992; Roncoroni *et al.* 1999), many other studies have suggested the opposite, namely that patients diagnosed soon after the onset of their symptoms have poorer outcomes (Macdonald 1951; Copeland *et al.* 1968; Pescatori *et al.* 1982; McDermott *et al.* 1981a, 1981b; Polissar *et al.* 1981; Schillaci *et al.* 1984; Chapuis *et al.* 1985; Barillari *et al.* 1989; Mulcahy & O'Donoghue 1997; Baig *et al.* 1999a). This is thought to result from 'biological predeterminism' (Macdonald 1951, 1958; Feinstein 1966) which proposes that aggressive cancers present with aggressive symptoms, resulting in earlier referral, diagnosis and treatment, whereas patients with less aggressive cancers present with more subtle symptoms, resulting in late referral and treatment. The effect of the biological nature of colorectal cancer on its symptomatic presentation may explain why the considerable efforts to achieve greater public awareness of the symptoms of bowel cancer and referral guidelines for GPs have made very little difference to reducing the 10–20% of cancer patients still having delays in referral and treatment of over a year (Tamoney & Caldarelli 1966; McSherry *et al.* 1969; Clarke & Jones 1970; Bassett *et al.* 1979; Turnbull & Isbister 1979; Polissar *et al.* 1981; Jolly *et al.* 1982; Khubchandani 1985; Barillari *et al.* 1989).

This effect of 'biological predeterminism' may, however, be obscuring a benefit of earlier symptomatic diagnosis in a small number of patients in studies of this nature. To attempt to avoid this paradoxical effect, the effect of delay after the hospital outpatient appointment on survival was studied on the assumption that delays after this point in the cancer patient's journey would more likely be caused by random clinical and administrative factors, and not just the biological nature of the cancer. This study still showed no evidence of poorer clinical outcomes even in patients having hospital delays in treatment of over 5 months (Baig *et al.* 1999b).

Although these observational studies have potentially serious biases, which may obscure some small benefit of earlier symptomatic diagnosis and treatment, the overall evidence suggests that a large proportion of patients die from cancer in spite of prompt treatment, and a substantial number survive in spite of prolonged delays in treatment (Baig *et al.* 1999c). This suggests that the critical point at which most cancers change from being curable to incurable occurs either before the minimum time that can be achieved to treatment or long after this point in time.

It is axiomatic that only patients with cancers having a critical point within 1 or 2 months after the minimum achievable time to treatment, and who at the moment are treated after this point in time, could benefit from earlier symptomatic diagnosis.

The evidence so far therefore suggests that the benefit in terms of overall better survival of all patients with colorectal cancer by policies aiming to achieve prompt referral and investigation of all patients with lower GI symptoms is likely to be small (Keddie & Hargreaves 1968; Slaney 1971; Holliday & Hardcastle 1979; McDermott *et al.* 1981a, 1981b; Goodman & Irvin 1993; Irvin & Greaney 1997; Baig *et al.* 1999a). This small possible theoretical benefit has to be balanced against the disadvantage of investigating very large numbers of patients without cancer.

Summary of the basis for a new paradigm governing the investigation of patients with lower GI symptoms

- The high prevalence of lower GI symptoms in the community and in general practice, and their low predictive value for cancer, establish the need for a policy of selection.
- The failure of studies to demonstrate a benefit of earlier symptomatic diagnosis strongly supports the conclusion that short time lags before referral do little harm.
- 'Treat, watch and wait' strategies, which are already being used by patients in the community and by GPs in primary care, are safe as well as prudent, even though this will inevitably result in a time lag or 'delay' of variable length in referral and treatment of patients with cancer.
- The challenge for referral guidelines is to define criteria, which identify patients at higher and low risk of cancer, and to assign appropriate 'waits' in 'treat, watch and wait' policies according to cancer risk.

- In primary care, estimates of cancer risk have to be based on age, symptom patterns, a simple clinical examination and haemoglobin estimation.
- Patients presenting with low-risk symptoms will need to understand that the longer time lags before referral are appropriate to avoid over-investigation of patients without cancer.

The next part of this chapter summarises how the criteria for estimating cancer risk have been identified.

The common symptom and sign patterns of patients with established cancer

It is likely that the common symptom and sign patterns in established cancer will have higher predictive and diagnostic value. Until recently it has been reported that the presenting symptoms of patients with colorectal cancer are indistinguishable from patients with piles or irritable bowel syndrome (Keddie & Hargreaves 1968; Curless *et al*. 1994). It has also been assumed that the early symptoms of colorectal cancer are even less specific (Holliday & Hardcastle 1979; MacAdam 1979). These ideas are based on studies of the prevalence of single primary symptoms of bowel cancer independently of the other important and commonly associated diagnostic factors (Keddie & Hargreaves 1968; McSherry 1969; Bassett *et al*. 1979; Turnbull & Isbister 1979; Polissar *et al*. 1981; Jolly *et al*. 1982; Pescatori *et al*. 1982; Schillaci *et al*. 1984; Curless *et al*. 1994; Mulcahy & O'Donoghue 1997). However, it is clear from the same studies that many patients must present with combinations of symptoms and signs, and it is likely that these will have higher predictive and diagnostic value than the individual symptoms or signs alone.

Previous studies have also shown the clear difference between the mode of presentation and symptom patterns of rectal and sigmoid cancers as compared with more proximal cancers. For example, 55–65% of distal cancers present with both rectal bleeding and a change in bowel habit, and only 20–25% present with a change in bowel habit alone and 15–20% with rectal bleeding alone (Dodds *et al*. 1999; Doueck *et al*. 1999; Ellis *et al*. 1999a, 1999b). Most of the latter patients are relatively easy to distinguish from patients with piles because up to 60% have no anal symptoms (Dodds *et al*. 1999; Ellis *et al*. 1999a, 1999b), and 40–50% will have a palpable anorectal mass (Holliday & Hardcastle 1979; Goodman & Irvin 1993; Ellis *et al*. 1999a). In one study only 3% of patients presenting with rectal bleeding from rectal and sigmoid cancers had symptoms indistinguishable from piles (Dodds *et al*. 1999).

In contrast to these patients, half of the cancers proximal to the sigmoid have a significant iron deficiency anaemia at presentation, 40% have a palpable abdominal mass and up to a third present as an emergency with intestinal obstruction (Keddie & Hargreaves 1968; Bassett *et al*. 1979; Chapuis *et al*. 1985; Ellis *et al*. 1999a) often with short histories. Only 5% of patients with proximal cancers present with a change in bowel habit and/or abdominal pain without these other additional diagnostic factors (Ellis *et al.* 1999a).

The nature of the change in bowel habit is also important, with 80–90% of all cancer patients with this symptom having increased frequency of defecation and/or increased looseness of their stools (Dodds *et al.* 1999; Ellis *et al.* 1999a).

The higher predictive and diagnostic value of symptom combinations compared with individual symptoms

Recent studies in primary (Fijten *et al.* 1995; Metcalf *et al.* 1996; Ellis *et al.* 1999b) and secondary care (Dodds *et al.* 1999) have shown the significantly higher predictive and diagnostic value of rectal bleeding when this occurs in association with a change in bowel habit or without anal symptoms (Table 12.2). Although the characteristics of rectal bleeding have long been thought to be of value, there is little evidence of this apart from dark-red bleeding (Metcalf *et al.* 1996; Ellis *et al.* 1999b; Chave *et al.* 2000) (Table 12.2).

The low predictive and diagnostic value of abdominal pain

Two studies in general practice showed that the presence of abdominal pain in patients with rectal bleeding and a change in bowel habit reduce the probability of cancer (Fitjen *et al.* 1995; Ellis *et al.* 1999b), whereas a third showed that it was of diagnostic value for serious disease (Metcalf *et al.* 1996). In a hospital study (Dodds *et al.* 1999), abdominal pain in association with the symptom combination of rectal bleeding/change in bowel habit significantly decreased the probability of cancer and, when it occurred without other symptoms as a single symptom, an unusual presentation, the risk of cancer was also significantly decreased (Dodds *et al.* 1999).

The effect of age on the predictive value of symptoms and symptom patterns in colorectal cancer

Of all colorectal cancers 1.5% occur below the age of 40 and 85% over the age of 60 (Cancer Research Campaign 1999). There is a steep rise in prevalence between the ages of 55 and 65 (Cancer Research Campaign 1999). This means that, for any symptom or symptom pattern, age will have a considerable effect on its predictive and diagnostic value. In one large study in a surgical outpatient clinic, the prevalence of cancer varied from 1:2 in patients over the age of 80 having the symptom pattern with the highest predictive value to 1:900 in patients below the age of 50 with the symptom and sign pattern with the lowest predictive value (Dodds *et al.* 1999) (Table 12.3).

It is clearly sensible to have different speeds of referral for patients with such large differences in cancer risk, with higher-risk patients being promptly referred and low-risk ones only referred after longer periods of 'treat, watch and wait'.

Table 12.2 The predictive and diagnostic value of the symptom combinations of rectal bleeding and when the rectal bleeding is described as dark red

	Reference	Sensitivity (%)	(%)	PPV (%)	LR (%)	95%CI	PPV without a change in bowel habit (%)
Rectal bleeding with a change in bowel habit	Fijten et al. (1995)	88.9	78.0	10.7	4.0	2.9–5.5	0.4
	Ellis et al. (1999b)[a]	100	57.6	9.2	2.4	1.6–2.7	0
	Dodds et al. (1999)	75.2	64.6	12.7	2.13	2.0–2.3	2.5
							PPV with anal symptoms (%)
Rectal bleeding without anal symptoms	Ellis et al. (1999b)[a]	63.6	78.0	11.1	2.9	1.6–4.3	2.0
	Dodds et al. (1999)	59.4	73.3	13.2	2.2	2.0–2.5	3.6
							PPV of bright red bleeding
Dark-red bleeding	Ellis et al. (1999b)[a]	27.3	88.1	9.4	2.3	0.8–5.3	3.6
	Metcalf et al. (1996)	37.5	70.0	11.1	1.25	0.5–3.2	8.2
	Chave et al. (2000)	36.5	82.5	12.7	2.08	1.8–2.5	5.1

[a]Hospital population.
95%CI, 95% confidence interval; LR, likelihood ratio = sensitivity/(1 – specificity); PPV, positive predictive value.

Table 12.3 The effect of age on the prevalence of cancer in patients with various symptom patterns in a surgical outpatient clinic

Age (years)	All patients with rectal bleeding	All patients with both rectal bleeding and a change in bowel habit	All patients who presented with both rectal bleeding and a change in bowel habit, but no abdominal pain or perianal symptoms	All patients presenting with rectal bleeding without a change in bowel habit and without perianal symptoms	All patients presenting with rectal bleeding without a change in bowel habit and with perianal symptoms[a]	All patients with a change in bowel habit and no rectal bleeding	All patients with abdominal pain without rectal bleeding and without a change in bowel habit
Total number of patients	5,442	2,063	331	810	2,544	1,845	655
Nos of cancers	347	261	97	49	16	110	16
<39	1:268	1:73	1:26	1:148	0.633	1:97	0:71
40–49	1:83	1:32	1:9	1:122	1:255	1:79	1:93
50–59	1:26	1:13	1:6	1:62	1:178	1:25	1:25
60–69	1:10	1:6	1:3	1:13	1:100	1:22	1:41
70–79	1:8	1:6	1:3	1:8	1:47	1:10	1:36
≥80	1:5	1:4	1:2	1:6	1:18	1:14	1:21
Total	**1:16**	**1:8**	**1:3**	**1:17**	**1:159**	**1:17**	**1:41**

[a]Not including patients with a palpable rectal mass or abdominal mass or patients with an iron deficiency anaemia < 10 g.

The predictive value of an iron deficiency anaemia for colorectal cancer

The predictive value of an iron deficiency anaemia (IDA) for cancer in primary care is unknown, but it is likely to vary with age, the level of haemoglobin, and according to the presence or absence of the primary symptoms of colorectal cancer. However, all levels of IDA, even without symptoms and signs, particularly in elderly people, must be treated seriously and, even if mild, investigation must be considered. Of cancer patients presenting with an IDA, 50% do not have any symptoms or signs. The haemoglobin is < 10 g in most patients presenting with anaemia from a colorectal cancer by the time they present (Tamoney & Caldarelli 1966; Wright & Higgins 1982; Fegiz *et al.* 1989; Goodman & Irvin 1993), and it is likely that levels below this will have a higher predictive value than a mild IDA, which is relatively common in elderly people.

The diagnostic value of faecal occult blood examinations in symptomatic patients for colorectal cancer

The Haemoccult test is of little diagnostic value in symptomatic patients in hospital (Goulston & Davidson 1980; Leicester *et al.* 1983) and of no proven value in symptomatic patients in primary care.

The diagnostic value of a positive family history for cancer and significant polyps in symptomatic patients

There is little information on the value of a positive family history in symptomatic patients (Chapuis *et al.* 1985; Nichols *et al.* 1999). It is particularly important in the management of patients with low-risk symptoms (Chapuis *et al.* 1985; Nichols *et al.* 1999) to know whether the possible increase in risk is sufficient for them to be referred to a fast-track clinic.

Determination of the higher-risk criteria for referral on the basis of the '2-week standard'

The challenge for providing advice for public awareness campaigns and the new referral guidelines is to identify criteria determining cancer risk that maintain high sensitivity for cancer, i.e. include the majority of patients with cancer with as little loss of specificity as possible, by reducing the numbers of patients with benign disease needing investigation.

It is important to understand that 'as sensitivity increases, a point is reached at which very small increases in sensitivity are accompanied by very large decreases in specificity i.e. the number of false-positive results increases. An increase in the number of false-positive test results increases patient anxiety, the costs of "investigation" and the risk associated with unnecessary "investigation"' (Muir Gray 1997b):

Sensitivity increases
↓
Specificity decreases
↓
Costs, risk and patient anxiety increase

The implication of this for the referral guidelines is that there will be an exponential increase in the number of patients needing to be investigated to capture the last few cancer patients with less common and low-risk presentations.

In a study of over 8,000 surgical outpatients (Dodds *et al.* 1999), the cumulative percentage of cancers diagnosed was plotted against the cumulative percentage of all patients examined for each of nine symptom patterns in patients above and below the age of 60 ranked according to increasing diagnostic yields (Figure 12.1). This showed that proportionately more patients need to be investigated for each cancer detected as the diagnostic yield decreases. Using the age and symptom profiles with predictive values down to 5.4% (as1–as9; Figure 12.1), 83% of cancer patients were diagnosed by examining 39% of all patients with these symptoms. Thus, the overall sensitivity of this group of age and symptom profiles was 83% (as1–as9) with a false-positive rate of 39%.

The Guidelines Committee decided the Government's new '2-week standard' for bowel cancer could be achieved with little increase in existing resources using age and symptom profiles with a positive predictive value of not less than 5%, based on hospital data. It was accepted that the same age and symptom profiles in primary care will have a lower diagnostic yield, which will result in a larger number of patients needing to be investigated for each cancer detected.

The Department of Health's recommendations for referral guidelines for bowel cancer

It was recommended that the age and symptom profiles listed below *when occurring for the first time*, not as a recurrent episode, persistent for at least 6 weeks and together with signs where appropriate and an iron deficiency anaemia (IDA), should be used to identify patients for referral on the basis of the government's new '2-week standard'. It has been estimated that the higher-risk criteria should identify 80–90% of patients with bowel cancer presenting to GPs, while keeping to a minimum the number of patients without cancer needing to be referred to the fast-track system (Table 12.4).

It is equally important to emphasise the importance of identifying patients at very low risk of cancer, who can be safely treated for longer periods in primary care. The low-risk criteria are listed in Table 12.5.

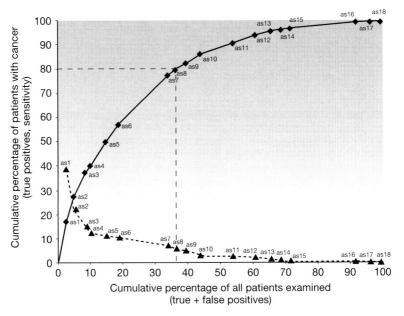

Figure 12.1

Key to Figure 12.1

Symptoms	Cumulative % of Cancer patients	All patients	Diagnostic value for cancer (%)
as1	17.2	2.5	38.9
as2	27.1	5.0	22.4
as3	36.8	8.6	15.3
as4	39.9	10.0	12.5
as5	49.8	14.8	11.5
as6	57.4	18.8	10.9
as7	77.3	33.9	7.5
as8	80.0	36.4	6.1
as9	83.0	39.4	5.4
as10	85.5	43.9	3.2
as11	90.8	53.9	3.0
as12	93.9	60.7	2.6
as13	95.6	65.7	1.9
as14	96.4	68.9	1.4
as15	96.8	71.6	0.9
as16	99.4	92.1	0.7
as17	99.7	96.8	0.5
as18	100.0	100.0	0.4

Key to symptom and age graph

Symptoms	Age ≥60 years	<60 years
+C +B −PS −AP	as1	as4
+C +B −PS +AP	as2	as8
+C +B +PS −AP	as3	as9
+C +B +PS +AP	as6	as13
+C −B	as7	as12
−C +B −PS	as5	as17
−C −B +AP	as10	as14
−C +B +PS	as11	as16
−C −B −AP +PS	as15	as18

C = change in bowel habit; B = rectal bleeding; PS = perianal symptoms; AP = abdominal pain; '+' symptom present; '−' symptom absent.

For example, +C +B −PS −AP = patients with a change in bowel habit with rectal bleeding without perianal symptoms and abdominal pain.

Table 12.4 Higher-risk criteria

Criteria	Age threshold (years)
Rectal bleeding WITH a change in bowel habit to looser stools and/or increased frequency of defecation persistent for 6 weeks	All ages
Change in bowel habit as above without rectal bleeding and persistent for 6 weeks	> 60
Rectal bleeding persistently WITHOUT anal symptoms[a]	> 60
A definite palpable right-sided abdominal mass	All ages
A definite palpable rectal mass (not pelvic)	All ages

Unexplained iron deficiency anaemia
    Men < 11 g
    Women < 10 g
	
	All ages
	Postmenopausal

[a]Anal symptoms include soreness, discomfort, itching, lumps and prolapse as well as pain.

Table 12.5 Lower-risk criteria

Criteria	Age threshold
Rectal bleeding WITH anal symptoms	All ages
Rectal bleeding with an obvious external cause for the bleeding on simple examination of the perineum, e.g. anal fissure, a thrombosed or prolapsed pile, and rectal prolapse	All ages
Transient changes in bowel habit, particularly to harder stools and/or decreased frequency of defecation	All ages
Abdominal pain as a single symptom WITHOUT other higher-risk age/symptom/sign profiles, an abdominal mass, an iron deficiency anaemia or intestinal obstruction.	All ages

Management of patients with low-risk criteria

Approximately 10–20% of patients with colorectal cancer will present with low-risk symptom and sign patterns, and most of these patients will continue to be diagnosed in routine clinics. Careful 'treat, watch and wait' management strategies are therefore needed in primary care to avoid excessive time lags before referral of these low-risk patients if their symptoms persist. These strategies must be with the agreement of the patient, who will need to understand the overall benefit to the majority of patients without cancer of avoiding unnecessary investigations. Patients who are not happy with this arrangement can still be referred routinely to a normal clinic. Patients may have written information about higher-risk symptoms so they can self-refer back at an earlier stage if these develop as part of 'safety netting'. If patients are overly anxious with low-risk symptoms or in younger age groups with persistent higher-risk symptoms, i.e. rectal bleeding *without* anal symptoms, there is always a third alternative route for referral – *an urgent appointment in a routine clinic*. This mode of referral must be kept to a minimum, however, to ensure that all patients referred in this way are promptly seen. There are therefore three speeds of referral depending on cancer risk and the concern of the patient and the GP (Figure 12.2).

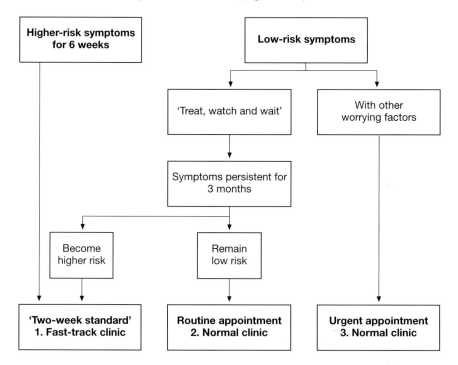

Figure 12.2 The three routes or speeds of referral.

Implications for service organisation

An estimate of the numbers of patients needing to be seen in outpatients each year on the basis of the '2-week standard' for a population of 100,000 was determined using the following assumptions and calculations:

- 58 new bowel cancers per 100,000 population per year (Cancer in the South-West 1999) of which 25% or 14 will present as an emergency, leaving 44 to be seen in the outpatient clinic (Wessex Colorectal Cancer Audit, 1999, personal communication)
- 90% of these 44 patients will have higher-risk symptoms = 40 patients
- the diagnostic yields in the fast-track clinics will be between 5% and 10% (Ellis *et al.* 1998; Dodds *et al.* 1999)
- this means 10–20 patients are seen for every cancer diagnosed, which will result in 400–800 patients needing investigation each year
- eight patients will be seen per clinic

- the number of clinics needed per year = (400 – 800)/8 = 50–100 clinics per year
- 42 clinics per year per doctor allowing for annual and study leave and other absences
- 50–100/42 = 1.1–2.2 clinics per week per 100,000 of the population per year
- assumes that the fast-track clinics will include all the higher-risk cancer patients diagnosed in outpatients. If only 50% of the higher-risk patients are referred to the fast-track clinics, the total number of patients needing to be seen in the fast-track clinic will be half of that predicted
- if all these patients are already being seen in normal clinics, a simple reconfiguration of the outpatient appointments is all that is necessary and there will be no need for extra clinics.

However, as there is already a problem with long waiting times for outpatient clinics in many districts, it was the view of the Referral Guidelines Drafting Committee and virtually all the reviewers of the document that the new government policy will increase the referral rate. There will therefore have to be a substantial increase in the number of clinics for these patients, if the '2-week standard' is to be achieved without greatly increasing the overall delay of all patients referred to hospital with lower gastrointestinal symptoms.

Summary

There will be a need for between 400 and 800 outpatient appointments per year or 1.1 to 2.2 clinics per week per 100,000 of the population, assuming 100% effectiveness (all cancer patients with higher-risk symptoms referred to these clinics) of the Guidelines.

Estimation of number of barium enema requests likely to arise from patients seen in the fast-track system

The rate of ordering a barium enema following flexible sigmoidoscopy in a colorectal clinic varied from 5% to 25% (Dodds & Thompson 1993; Ellis *et al.* 1998). Taking the average figure of 15% and assuming that 400–800 patients will be seen per year per 100,000 of the population on the basis of the '2-week standard', this will result in 60–120 requests for barium enemas each year. Ring-fenced resources should be provided for at least this number of examinations (2–3 per week per 100,000 of the population), which should be done within the standard time set locally.

In hospitals where investigation of these patients is initially by rigid sigmoidoscopy, substantially more patients will need a barium enema or colonoscopy examination.

Estimation of the numbers of patients likely to need colonoscopy as a result of referrals on the basis of the '2-week standard'

On the basis that 10% of patients will have adenomatous polyps (Dodds *et al*. 1998) and that all of these will go forward for colonoscopy, this will require 40–80 colonoscopies per 100,000 of the population per year (0.8–1.6 per 100,000 population per week). Ring-fenced resources should be provided for these colonoscopies to be done within the standard set locally. If colonoscopy is used for diagnosis, considerably more will need to be done.

Effective dissemination of the guidelines

The implementation of guidelines is complex and problematic, and merely devising accurate and up-to-date evidence-based guidelines and even presenting them attractively is unlikely to ensure that they will be implemented. The conventional forms of continuing education, unsolicited written communication or oral communication through lectures have been shown to be ineffective in changing doctors' practice. GPs are a diverse group of doctors whose response to implementation and strategy is not uniform, so multiple strategies are essential for successful implementation. The Department of Health referral guidelines made specific recommendations from the literature on the implementation of guidelines and suggested the following practical strategies, which have been shown to be effective and support previous theoretical analyses on professional judgement and decision-making by GPs:

- The development within a general practice of 'an evaluative culture' (Haines & Jones 1994), including regular audit of practice and 'critical incident' analysis (Allery *et al*. 1997).
- Continuing education based on and reflecting the practice of GPs (Cantillon & Jones 1999).
- Peer review and group learning (Wensing *et al*. 1998).
- Personal education development plans that prompts GPs into seeing that they have a specific educational need, which they might not yet have recognised (Tracey *et al*. 1997).
- Organisational and management support is essential (Dubin 1990) involving consideration of work assignments, interactions of colleagues, feedback and reward structure (Grimshaw & Ryssell 1993).
- The local development of guidelines (Dubin 1990), e.g. local groups developing their own guidelines based on nationally agreed ones but incorporating local practice and conditions.
- Local outreach visits from opinion leaders (Davis *et al*. 1995).
- Follow-up 're-education' at regular intervals to reinforce GPs' learning (Rutz *et al*. 1991).

- Personalised feedback, e.g. from a hospital specialist to a particular GP (Winkens *et al.* 1992; O'Connell *et al.* 1999).
- Computer prompts during a GP's consultation with a patient (Johnstone *et al.* 1994; Lobach 1996).

Conclusion

The long delays in treatment of a small, but significant, number of patients with colorectal cancer is unacceptable and has not changed for at least 50 years in spite of public awareness campaigns and referral guidelines for primary care doctors. It is now possible that the identification of age/symptom/sign profiles identifying patients at higher or low risk of cancer with different speeds of referral and better management of an iron deficiency anaemia will significantly increase the effectiveness and efficiency of diagnosis of bowel cancer. This will greatly improve the quality of care of many cancer patients, and may increase the chance of survival of those who at present experience long delays before referral. The referral guidelines should also increase the quality of care of many patients without cancer by safely avoiding the unnecessary worry of hospital referral and investigation, particularly those with transient or intermittent, low-risk symptoms.

However, it has to be emphasised that many patients with persistent low-risk symptoms will still need investigation because they will include up to 15% of all patients with bowel cancer. This means that, even with highly efficient management of all patients with lower gastrointestinal symptoms, large numbers of patients will still need investigation, and prompt diagnosis of *all* patients with colorectal cancer, not just those with higher risk symptom/sign profiles, will not be achieved without a substantial increase in resources.

> The fundamental aim of the referral guidelines is not to determine whether a patient should be referred for investigation, but to advise on the speed of referral so that those at higher risk are seen promptly and those at low risk have longer periods of 'watchful waiting', enabling patients with minor, intermittent or transient symptoms to avoid investigation in hospital.

References

Allery L, Owen PA, Robling MR (1997). Why general practitioners and consultants change clinical practice: a critical incident study. *British Medical Journal* **314**, 870–874

Baig MK, Whatley P, Thompson MR (1999a). Delays during stages of referral diagnosis and treatment of colorectal cancer. Their relationship to mortality. *Colorectal Disease* **1**(suppl 1), 3.0.11

Baig MK, Whatley P, Thompson MR (1999b). Delay in diagnosis and treatment of colorectal cancer of colorectal cancer: Does it affect outcome? *Colorectal Disease* **1**(suppl 1), 3.0.10

Barillari P, de Angelis R, Valabrega S *et al*. (1989). Relationship of symptom duration and survival in patients with colorectal carcinoma. *European Journal of Surgical Oncology* **15**, 441–445

Bassett ML, Bennett SA, Goulston KJ (1979). Colorectal cancer. A study of 230 patients. *Medical Journal of Australia* 1, 589–592

Blakeborough A, Sheridan MB, Chapman AH (1997). Complications of Barium Enema Examinations: a Survey of UK Consultant Radiologists (1992 to (1994. *Clinical Radiology* **52**, 142–148

Byles JE, Redman S, Hennrikus D, Sanson-Fisher RW, Dickinson J (1992). Delay in consulting a medical practitioner about rectal bleeding. *Journal of Epidemiology and Community Health* **46**, 241–244

Cancer Research Campaign (1999). *Guidelines*. London: Cancer Research Campaign

Cancer in the South and West. (1999). Annual Report 1988–1996. South-West Cancer Intelligence unit. Bristol/Winchester

Cantillon P & Jones R (1999). Does continuing medical education in general practice make a difference? *British Medical Journal* **318**, 1276–1279

Chapuis PH, Dent OF, Fisher R *et al*. (1985). A multivariate analysis of clinical and pathological variables in prognosis after resection of large bowel cancer. *British Journal of Surgery* **72**, 698–702

Chave H, Flashman K, Cripps NPJ, Senapati A, Thompson MR (2000). The relative values of the characteristics of rectal bleeding in the diagnosis of colorectal cancer. *Colorectal Disease* **2**(suppl 1), 1.01

Clarke AM & Jones ISC (1970). Diagnostic accuracy and diagnostic delay in carcinoma of the large bowel. *New Zealand Medical Journal* **71**, 341–347

Clarke JP, Kettlewell MGW, Dehn TCB (1992). Changing patterns of colorectal cancer in a regional teaching hospital. *Annals of the Royal College of Surgeons of England* **74**, 291–293

Connell AM, Hilton C, Irvine G, Lennard-Jones JE, Misiewicz J (1965). Variation of bowel habit in two population samples. *British Medical Journal* **ii**, 1095–1099

Copeland EM, Miller LD, Jones RS (1968). Prognostic factors in carcinoma of the colon and rectum. *American Journal of Surgery* **116**, 875–881

Crosland A & Jones R (1995). Rectal bleeding. Prevalence and consultation behaviour. *British Medical Journal* **311**, 486–488

Curless F, French J, Williams GV, James OFW (1994). Comparison of gastrointestinal symptoms in colorectal carcinoma patients and community controls with respect to age. *Gut* **35**, 1267–1270

Davis D, Thomson A, Oxman AD, Haynes RB (1995). Changing physician performance: A systematic review of the effect of continuing medical education strategies. *Journal of the American Medical Association* **274**, 700–705

Dent OF, Goulston KJ, Zubrzychi J, Chapuis PH (1986). Bowel symptoms in an apparently well population. *Diseases of the Colon and Rectum* **29**, 243–247

Dodds SR & Thompson MR (1993). Barium enema audit in a colorectal out-patients. *Gut* **34**(suppl 1), S27

Dodds SR & Thompson MR (1997). The value of a negative flexible sigmoidoscopy in surgical out-patients. *Gut* **40**(suppl 1), F261

Dodds SR, Baig K, Flashman K, Thompson MR, Senapati A (1998). a differences of barium enema following a normal out-patient flexible sigmoidoscopy: a case for audit? *Colorectal Disease* **15**(suppl 1), P57

Dodds S, Dodds A, Vakis S *et al.* (1999). The value of various factors associated with rectal bleeding in the diagnosis of colorectal cancer. *Gut* **44**, A99

Donald IP, Smith RG, Cruikshank JG, Elton RA, Stoddard ME (1985). A study of constipation in the elderly living at home. *Gerontology* **31**, 112–118

Douek M, Wickramasinghe M, Clifton MA (1999). Does isolated rectal bleeding suggest colorectal cancer? *The Lancet* **354**, 393

Drossman DA, Sandler RS, McKee DC, Lovitz AJ (1982). Bowel patterns among subjects not seeking health care. use of a questionnaire to identify a population with bowel dysfunction. *Gastroenterology* **83**, 112–118

Dubin SS (1990). Maintaining competence through updating. In Willis SL & Dubin SS (eds) *Maintaining Professional Competence*. San Francisco: Jossey Bass, pp 9–43

Ellis BG, Jones M, Senapati A, Golding P, Thompson MR (1998). Restricted but rapid access sigmoidoscopy clinic – is it the way forward? *Gut* **42**(suppl 1), T390

Ellis B, Baig MK, Cripps NPJ *et al.* (1999a). Common modes of presentation of colorectal cancer patients. *Colorectal Disease* **1**(suppl 1), 24

Ellis BG, Jones M, Thompson MR (1999b). Rectal bleeding in general practice: who needs referral? *Colorectal Disease* **1**(suppl 1), 23–24

Everhart JE, Go VLW, Johannes RS, Fitzsimmons SC, Roth HP, White LR (1989). A longitudinal survey of self-reported bowel habits in the United States. *Digestive Disease Science* **34**, 1153–1162

Farrands PA & Hardcastle JD (1984). Colorectal screening by a self-completion questionnaire. *Gut* **25**, 445–447

Fegiz G, Barillari P, Ramacciato G *et al.* (1989). Right colon cancer: long-term results after curative surgery and prognostic significance of duration of symptoms. *Journal of Surgical Oncology* **41**, 250–255

Feinstein AR (1966). Symptoms as an index of biological behaviour and prognosis in human cancer. *Nature* **209**, 241–245

Fijten G, Blijham GH, Knottnerus JA (1994). Occurrence and clinical significance of overt blood loss per rectum in the general population and in medical practice. A review. *British Journal of General Practice* **44**, 320–325

Fijten GH, Starmans R, Muris JWM, Schouten HJA, Blijham GH, Knottnerus JA (1995). Predictive value of signs and symptoms for colorectal cancer in patients with rectal bleeding in general practice. *Family Practitioner* **12**, 279–286

Goodman D & Irvin TT (1993). Delay in the diagnosis and prognosis of carcinoma of the right colon. *British Journal of Surgery* **80**, 1327–1329

Goulston KJ & Davidson P (1980). Faecal occult blood testing in patients with colonic symptoms. *Medical Journal of Australia* **2**, 667–668

Grimshaw JM & Russell IT (1993). Effect of clinical guidelines on medical practice: a systematic review of rigorous evaluations. *The Lancet* **342**, 1317–1322

Haines A & Jones R (1994). Implementing Research Findings. *British Medical Journal* **308**, 1488–1490

Hannay DR (1979). *The Symptom Iceberg: A study of Community Health*. London: Routledge & Kegan Paul

Hardcastle JD, Chamberlain JO, Robinson MHE *et al.* (1996). Randomised control trial of faecal occult blood screening for colorectal cancer. *The Lancet* **348**, 1472–1477

Haynes RB, Sackett DL, Taylor DW, Gibson ES, Johnson AL (1978). Increased absenteeism from work after detection and labeling of hypertensive patients. *New England Journal of Medicine* **299**, 741–744

Heaton KW, O'Donnell LJD, Braddon FEM, Mountford RA, Hughes AO, Cripps PJ (1992a). Symptoms of irritable bowel syndrome in a British urban community. consulters and non-consulters. *Gastroenterology* **102**, 1962–1967

Heaton KW, Radvan J, Cripps H, Mountford RA, Braddon FEM, Hughes AO (1992b). Defecation frequency and timing, and stool form in the general population. a prospective study. *Gut* **33**, 529–534

Holliday HW & Hardcastle JD (1979). Delay in diagnosis and treatment of symptoms colorectal cancer. *The Lancet* **i**, 309–311

Irvin TT & Greaney MG (1997). Duration of symptoms and prognosis of carcinoma of the colon and rectum. *Surgical Gynecology and Obstetrics* **144**, 883–886

Johnstone ME, Langton KB, Haynes RB (1994). Effects of computer-based clinical decision support systems on clinical performances and patient outcome. *Archives of Internal Medicine* **120**, 135–142

Jolly KD, Scott JP, MacKinnon MJ, Clarke AM (1982). Diagnosis and survival in carcinoma of the large bowel. *Australia New Zealand Journal of Surgery* **52**, 12–16

Jones ISC (1976). An analysis of bowel habit and its significance in the diagnosis of carcinoma of the colon. *American Journal of Proctology* **27**, 45–46

Jones R & Lydeard S (1992). Irritable bowel syndrome in the general population. *British Medical Journal* **303**, 87–90

Kay L, Jorgensen T, Schultz-Larsen K (1992). Abdominal pain in a 70 year-old Danish population. An epidemiological study of the prevalence and importance of abdominal pain. *Journal of Clinical Epidemiology* **45**, 1377–1382

Keddie N & Hargreaves A (1968). Symptoms of carcinoma of the colon and rectum. *The Lancet* **ii** 749–750

Kewenter J, Haglind E, Smith L (1989). Value of a risk questionnaire in screening for colorectal neoplasm. *British Journal of Surgery* **76**, 280–283

Khubchandani M (1985). Relationship of symptom duration and survival in patients and carcinoma of the colon and rectum. *Diseases of the Colon and Rectum* **28**, 585–587

Kronborg O, Fenger C, Olsen J, Jorgensen OD, Sandegaard O (1996). Randomised study of screening for colorectal cancer with faecal occult blood test. *The Lancet* **348**, 1467–1471

Launoy G, Le Courtour X, Gignoux M, Pottier D, Dugleux G (1992). Influence of rural environment on diagnosis, treatment and prognosis of colorectal cancer. *Journal of Epidemiology and Community Health* **46**, 365–367

Leicester RJ, Lightfoot A, Millar J, Colin Jones DG, Hunt RH (1983). Accuracy and value of the Haem occult test in symptomatic patients. *British Medical Journal* **286**, 673–674

Lobach DF (1996). Electronically distributed, computer-generated, individualized feedback enhances the use of computerized practice guideline. *Proceedings of the American Medical Informatics Association annual fall symposium*, pp 493–497

MacAdam DB (1979). A study in general practice of the symptoms and delay patterns in the diagnosis of gastrointestinal cancer. *Journal of the Royal College of General Practitioners* **29**, 723–729

MacArthur C & Smith A (1984). Factors associated with speed of diagnosis, referral and treatment in colorectal cancer. *Journal of Epidemiology and Community Health* **38**, 122–126

Macdonald I (1951). Biological predeterminism in human cancer. *Surgical Gynecology and Obstetrics* **92**, 443–452

Macdonald I (1958). The individual basis of biologic variability in cancer. *Surgical Gynecology and Obstetrics* **106**, 227–229

MacDonald LA, Sackett DL, Haynes RB, Taylor DW (1984). Labelling in hypertension: A review of the behavioural and psychological consequences. *Journal of Chronic Diseases* **37**, 933–942

McDermott F, Hughes E, Pihl E, Milne B, Price A (1981a). Symptom duration and survival prospects in carcinoma of the rectum. *Surgical Gynecology and Obstetrics* **153**, 321–326

McDermott FT, Hughes ESR Pihl E, Milnes BJ, Price AB (1981b). Prognosis in relation to symptom duration in colon cancer. *British Journal of Surgery* **68**, 846–849

McSherry CK, Cornell GN, Glenn F (1969). Carcinoma of the colon and rectum. *Annals of Surgery* **169**, 502–509

Mandel J, Church T, Ederer F, Bond J (1999). colorectal cancer mortality: effectiveness of biennial screening for fecal occult blood. *Journal of the National Cancer Institute* **91**, 434–437

Marshall KG (1996). Prevention. How much harm? How much benefit? 3. Physical psychological and social harm. *Canadian Medical Association* **155**, 169–176

Metcalf JV, Smith J, Jones R, Record CO (1996). Incidence and causes of rectal bleeding in general practice as detected by colonoscopy. *British Journal of General Practice* **46**, 161–164

Milne JS & Williamson J (1972). Bowel habit in older people. *Gerontological Clinics* **14**, 55–60

Muir Gray JA (1997a). Assessing the outcomes found. In: *Evidence-based Healthcare: How to make health policy and management decisions*, Chapter 6. Edinburgh: Churchill Livingstone

Muir Gray JA (1997b). Making decisions about health services. In*: Evidence-based Healthcare: How to make health policy and management decisions*, Chapter 3. Edinburgh: Churchill Livingstone, p 39

Mulcahy HE & O'Donoghue DP (1997). Duration of colorectal cancer symptoms and survival: the effect of confounding clinical and pathological variables. *European Journal of Cancer* **33**, 1461–1467

Muris JWM, Starmans R, Fijten GH, Crebolder HFJM, Krebber TFWA, Knottnerus JA (1993). Abdominal pain in general practice. *Family Practitioner* **10**, 387–390

Muris JWM, Starmans R, Fijten GH, Crebolder HFJM, Schouten HJA, Knottnerus JA (1995). Non-acute abdominal complaints in general practice: diagnostic value of signs and symptoms. *British Journal of General Practice* **45**, 313–316

Muris JWM, Starmans R, Fijten GH, Knottnerus JA (1996). One-year prognosis of abdominal complaints in general practice: a prospective study of patients in whom no organic cause is found. *British Journal of General Practice* **46**, 715–719

Neighbour R (1987). *The Inner Consultation. How to develop an effective and intuitive consulting style*. Lancaster: MTP Press Ltd (reprinted 1989, 1991)

Nichols PH, Cripps NPJ, Senapati A, Thompson MR (1999). Family history and colorectal cancer: A weak association in younger symptomatic patients. *Colorectal Disease* **1**(suppl 1), 23

O'Connell DL, Henry D, Tomlins R (1999). Randomised controlled trial of effect of feedback on general practitioners' prescribing in Australia. *British Medical Journal* **318**, 508–511

Pearse IH & Crocker LH (1985). *The Peckham Experiment. A study of the Living Structure of Society.* Scottish Edinburgh: Academic Press

Pescatori M, Maria G, Beltrani B, Mattana C (1982). Site, emergency and duration of symptoms in the prognosis of colorectal cancer. *Diseases of the Colon and Rectum* **25**, 33–40

Polissar L, Sim D, Francis A (1981). Survival of colorectal cancer patients in relation to duration of symptoms and other prognostic factors. *Diseases of the Colon and Rectum* **24**, 364–369

Robinson E, Mohilever J, Zidan J, Sapir D (1986). Colorectal cancer. Incidence delay in diagnosis and stage of disease. *European Journal of Cancer and Clinical Oncology* **22**, 157–161

Roncoroni L, Pietra N, Violi V, Sarli L, Choua O, Peracchia A (1999). Delay in the diagnosis and outcome of colorectal cancer: a prospective study. *European Journal of Surgical Oncology* **25**, 173–178

Rowe-Jones D & Aylett S (1965). Delay in treatment in carcinoma of colon and rectum *The Lancet* **ii**, 973–976

Rubin M, Zer M, Dintsman M (1980). Factors influencing delay in treatment of cancer of rectum and colon in Israel. *Israel Journal of Medical Science* **16**, 641–645

Rutz W, Von Knorring L, Walinder J (1991). Long-term effects of an educational program for general practitioners given by the Swedish committee for the prevention and treatment of depression. *Acta Psychiatrica Scandinavica* **85**, 83–88

Sackett DL, Haynes RB, Guyatt GH, Tugwell P (1991). Clinical diagnostic strategies. In: *Clinical Epidemiology – A basic science for clinical medicine*, 2nd edn, Chapter 1. London: Little Brown & Co., p 4

Sandler RS (1990). Epidemiology of irritable bowel syndrome in the United States. *Gastroenterology* **99**, 409–415

Sandler RS & Drossman DA (1987). Bowel habits in young adults not seeking health care. *Digestive Disease Science* **32**, 841–845

Schillaci A, Cavallaro A, Nicolanti V, Ferri M, Gallo P, Stipa S (1984). The importance of symptom duration in relation to prognosis of carcinoma of the large intestine. *Surgical Gynecology and Obstetrics* **158**, 423–426

Silman AJ, Mitchell P, Nicholls RJ *et al.* (1983). Self-reported dark red bleeding as a marker comparable with occult blood testing in screening for large bowel neoplasms. *British Journal of Surgery* **70**, 721–724

Slaney G (1971). Results of treatment of carcinoma of the colon and rectum. In Irvine WT (ed.) *Modern Trends in Surgery 3.* Sevenoaks: Butterworths, pp 69–89

Sonnenberg A & Koch TR (1989). Epidemiology of constipation in the United States. *Diseases of the Colon and Rectum* **32**, 1–8

Stewart-Brown S & Farmer A (1997). Screening could seriously damage your health. *British Medical Journal* **314**, 533–535

Talley NJ & Jones M (1998). Self-reported rectal bleeding in a United States community: prevalence, risk factors, and health care seeking. *American Journal of Gastroenterology* **11**, 2179–2183

Tamoney HJ Jr & Caldarelli RA (1966). Cancer of the right colon. an analysis of 211 patients. *Diseases of the Colon and Rectum* **9**(1), 13–19

Thompson JA, Pond CL, Ellis BG, Beach A, Thompson MR (2000). Rectal bleeding in general and hospital practice: 'The tip of the iceberg'. *Colorectal Disease* **2**, 288–293

Tracey J, Arroll B, Barham P, Richmond D (1997). The validity of general practitioners self-assessment of knowledge: cross sectional study. *British Medical Journal* **315**, 1426–1428

Turnbull PRG & Isbister WH (1979). Colorectal cancer in New Zealand: a Wellington study. *Australia New Zealand Journal of Surgery* **49**, 365–367

Wadsworth MEJ, Butterfield WJH, Blaney R (1971). *Health and Sickness, the Choice of Treatment. Perception of illness and use of services in an urban community.* London & Southampton: Tavistock Publications & Camelot Press Ltd

Waye JD (1995). Colonoscopy and proctosigmoidoscopy. In Haubrich W, Schaffner F, Berk JE (eds) *Bockus Gastroenterology*. Philadelphia: WB Saunders, p 323

Waye JD, Kahn O, Auerbach ME (1996). Complications of colonoscopy and flexible sigmoidoscopy. *Gastrointestinal Endoscopy Clinics of North America* **6**, 343–377

Welch CE & Burke JF (1962). Carcinoma of the colon and rectum. *New England Journal of Medicine* **266**, 846

Wensing M, Van Der Weijden T, Grol R (1998). Implementing guidelines and innovations in general practice: which interventions are effective? *British Journal of General Practice* **48**, 1–7

Williams CB (1986). Colonoscopy. *British Medical Bulletin* **42**, 265–269

Winkens R, Prop P, Grol R, Kester ADM, Knottnerus JA (1992). Effect of feedback on test ordering behaviour of general practitioners. *British Medical Journal* **304**, 1093–1096

Wright HK & Higgins EF (1982). Natural history of occult right colon cancer. *American Journal of Surgery* **143**, 169–170

Index